T0226895

Asthma in Childhood

Editors

LEONARD B. BACHARIER
THERESA W. GUILBERT

IMMUNOLOGY AND ALLERGY CLINICS OF NORTH AMERICA

www.immunology.theclinics.com

Consulting Editor
STEPHEN A. TILLES

May 2019 • Volume 39 • Number 2

ELSEVIER

1600 John F. Kennedy Boulevard • Suite 1800 • Philadelphia, Pennsylvania, 19103-2899
http://www.theclinics.com

IMMUNOLOGY AND ALLERGY CLINICS OF NORTH AMERICA Volume 39, Number 2
May 2019 ISSN 0889-8561, ISBN-13: 978-0-323-67787-5

Editor: Jessica McCool
Developmental Editor: Kristen Helm

Immunology and Allergy Clinics of North America (ISSN 0889–8561) is published quarterly by Elsevier Inc., 360 Park Avenue South, New York, NY 10010-1710. Months of issue are February, May, August, and November. Periodicals postage paid at New York, NY and additional mailing offices. Subscription prices are $341.00 per year for US individuals, $593.00 per year for US institutions, $100.00 per year for US students and residents, $423.00 per year for Canadian individuals, $220.00 per year for Canadian students, $753.00 per year for Canadian institutions, $447.00 per year for international individuals, $753.00 per year for international institutions, $220.00 per year for international students. To receive student/resident rate, orders must be accompanied by name of affiliated institution, date of term, and the *signature* of program/residency coordinator on institution letterhead. Orders will be billed at individual rate until proof of status is received. Foreign air speed delivery is included in all *Clinics* subscription prices. All prices are subject to change without notice. **POSTMASTER:** Send address changes to *Immunology and Allergy Clinics of North America*, Elsevier Health Sciences Division, Subscription Customer Service, 3251 Riverport Lane, Maryland Heights, MO 63043. **Customer Service: 1-800-654-2452 (U.S. and Canada); 314-447-8871 (outside U.S. and Canada). Fax:** 314-447-8029. **E-mail:** journalscustomerservice-usa@elsevier.com (for print support); journalsonlinesupport-usa@elsevier.com (for online support).

Reprints. For copies of 100 or more, of articles in this publication, please contact the Commercial Reprints Department, Elsevier Inc., 360 Park Avenue South, New York, New York 10010-1710. Tel. 212-633-3874, Fax: 212-633-3820, E-mail: reprints@elsevier.com.

Immunology and Allergy Clinics of North America is covered in MEDLINE/PubMed (Index Medicus), Current Contents/Life Sciences, Science Citation Index, ISI/BIOMED, Chemical Abstracts, and EMBASE/Excerpta Medica.

Contributors

CONSULTING EDITOR

STEPHEN A. TILLES, MD
Senior Director, Aimmune Therapeutics, Clinical Professor of Medicine, University of Washington, Seattle, Washington, USA

EDITORS

LEONARD B. BACHARIER, MD
Robert C. Strunk Endowed Chair for Lung and Respiratory Research, Professor of Pediatrics and Medicine, Edward Mallinckrodt Department of Pediatrics, Division of Allergy, Immunology, and Pulmonary Medicine, Washington University School of Medicine, St Louis, Missouri, USA

THERESA W. GUILBERT, MD, MS
Professor, Department of Pediatrics, University of Cincinnati, Pulmonary Division, Cincinnati Children's Hospital Medical Center, Cincinnati, Ohio, USA

AUTHORS

LEONARD B. BACHARIER, MD
Robert C. Strunk Endowed Chair for Lung and Respiratory Research, Professor of Pediatrics and Medicine, Edward Mallinckrodt Department of Pediatrics, Division of Allergy, Immunology, and Pulmonary Medicine, Washington University School of Medicine, St Louis, Missouri, USA

BRUCE G. BENDER, PhD
Professor of Pediatrics, Pediatric Behavioral Health, National Jewish Health, Denver, Colorado, USA

GENERY D. BOOSTER, PhD
Assistant Professor of Pediatrics, Pediatric Behavioral Health, National Jewish Health, Denver, Colorado, USA

AMAZIAH T. COLEMAN, MD
Division of Allergy and Immunology, Department of Pediatrics, Children's National Health System, George Washington University School of Medicine and Health Sciences, Washington, DC, USA

THERESA W. GUILBERT, MD, MS
Professor, Department of Pediatrics, University of Cincinnati, Pulmonary Division, Cincinnati Children's Hospital Medical Center, Cincinnati, Ohio, USA

SUJANI KAKUMANU, MD
Clinical Associate Professor, Department of Medicine, University of Wisconsin-Madison School of Medicine and Public Health, William S. Middleton Veterans Memorial Hospital, Madison, Wisconsin, USA

CAROLYN M. KERCSMAR, MD
Division of Pulmonary Medicine, Cincinnati Children's Hospital Medical Center, Cincinnati Children's Hospital, Cincinnati, Ohio, USA

CHRISTINA G. KWONG, MD
Assistant Professor, Department of Pediatrics, Washington University School of Medicine, St Louis, Missouri, USA

ROBERT F. LEMANSKE Jr, MD
Professor, Departments of Pediatrics and Medicine, Associate Dean for Clinical and Translational Research, Deputy Executive Director, Institute for Clinical and Translational Research, University of Wisconsin-Madison School of Medicine and Public Health, Madison, Wisconsin, USA

MARGEE LOUISIAS, MD, MPH
Division of Allergy and Immunology, Boston Children's Hospital, Harvard Medical School, Division of Rheumatology, Immunology and Allergy, Brigham and Women's Hospital, Boston, Massachusetts, USA

ANGELA MARKO, DO
Division of Pediatric Pulmonology, University Hospitals Rainbow Babies and Children's Hospital, Cleveland, Ohio, USA

FERNANDO D. MARTINEZ, MD
Regents Professor of Pediatrics, Asthma and Airways Disease Research Center, The University of Arizona, Tucson, Arizona, USA

KAREN M. McDOWELL, MD
Professor of Clinical Pediatrics, Division of Pulmonary Medicine, Cincinnati Children's Hospital Medical Center, Department of Pediatrics, University of Cincinnati College of Medicine, Cincinnati, Ohio, USA

AHMAD SALAHEDDINE NAJA, MD
Division of Allergy and Immunology, Boston Children's Hospital, Boston, Massachusetts, USA; Lebanese American University, Beirut, Lebanon, USA

ALYSSA A. OLAND, PhD
Assistant Professor of Pediatrics, Pediatric Behavioral Health, National Jewish Health, Denver, Colorado, USA

NATHAN M. PAJOR, MD
Clinical Fellow, Department of Pediatrics, Cincinnati Children's Hospital Medical Center, Cincinnati, Ohio, USA

WANDA PHIPATANAKUL, MD, MS
Division of Allergy and Immunology, Boston Children's Hospital, Harvard Medical School, Boston, Massachusetts, USA

BROOKE I. POLK, MD
Assistant Professor, Edward Mallinckrodt Department of Pediatrics, Division of Allergy, Immunology, and Pulmonary Medicine, Washington University in St. Louis, St Louis, Missouri, USA

AMIRA RAMADAN, MD
Division of Allergy and Immunology, Boston Children's Hospital, Beth Israel Deaconess Medical Center, Boston, Massachusetts, USA

KRISTIE R. ROSS, MD, MS
Division of Pediatric Pulmonology, University Hospitals Rainbow Babies and Children's Hospital, Associate Professor, Case Western Reserve University School of Medicine, Cleveland, Ohio, USA

WILLIAM J. SHEEHAN, MD
Division of Allergy and Immunology, Department of Pediatrics, Children's National Health System, George Washington University School of Medicine and Health Sciences, Washington, DC, USA

CASSIE SHIPP, MD
Clinical Pulmonary Fellow, Division of Pulmonary Medicine, Cincinnati Children's Hospital Medical Center, Cincinnati Children's Hospital, Cincinnati, Ohio, USA

STEPHEN J. TEACH, MD, MPH
George Washington University School of Medicine and Health Sciences, Division of Emergency Medicine, Department of Pediatrics, Children's National Health System, Washington, DC, USA

Contents

> Inappropriate responses to respiratory viruses, especially rhinovirus, and early allergic sensitization are the strongest contributors to the inception and persistence of early onset asthma. The ORMDL3 asthma locus in chromosome 17q seems to exert its effects by increasing susceptibility to human rhinovirus in early life. Being raised on animal farms is highly protective against the development of asthma, and this protective effect is mediated by exposure to microbes. Two trials in high-risk young children, one to prevent wheezing lower respiratory tract illness using bacterial lyophilizates and another using anti-immunoglobulin E to prevent asthma progression, are already under way.

> Asthma is the most common chronic disease of childhood in developed countries, with a continually increasing prevalence. The paradigm of asthma control is shifting from disease management to primary prevention, and the modification of numerous host and external factors have been proposed as methods to prevent recurrent wheeze and asthma in children, some with promising preliminary results. This article reviews potential asthma prevention strategies and identifies future areas of research.

> Asthma is highly prevalent and causes significant morbidity in children. The development of asthma depends on complex relationships between genetic predisposition and environmental modifiers of immune function. The biological and physical environmental factors include aeroallergens, microbiome, endotoxin, genetics, and pollutants. The psychosocial environment encompasses stress, neighborhood safety, housing, and discrimination. They all have been speculated to influence asthma control and the risk of developing asthma. Control of the factors that contribute to or aggravate symptoms, interventions to eliminate allergen exposure,

guidelines-based pharmacologic therapy, and education of children and their caregivers are of paramount importance.

The management of asthma in the preschool population is challenging because disease phenotypes are heterogeneous and evolving. Available therapies aimed at preventing persistent symptoms and recurrent exacerbations include inhaled corticosteroids and leukotriene receptor antagonists; episodic use of inhaled corticosteroids and azithromycin may result in a decrease in exacerbations among children with intermittent disease. This article reviews an approach using patient characteristics for selecting initial treatment approaches based on disease phenotype, such as symptom patterns or evidence of atopic markers. Evidence for and against the use of oral corticosteroids during acute episodes and barriers to adherence and effective treatment are discussed.

Asthma is a complex heterogeneous disease characterized by reversible airflow obstruction. After appropriate diagnosis, the management in school-aged children centers on 3 broad domains: pharmacologic treatment, treatment of underlying comorbidities, and education of the patient and caregivers. It is important to understand that the phenotypic differences that exist in the school-aged child with asthma may impact underlying comorbid conditions as well as pharmacologic treatment choices. Following initiation of therapy, asthma control must be continually evaluated in order to optimize management.

Objective measures of lung function are important in the diagnosis and management of asthma. Spirometry, the pulmonary function test most widely used in asthma, requires respiratory maneuvers that may be difficult for preschoolers. Impulse oscillometry (IOS) is a noninvasive method of measuring lung function during tidal breathing; hence, IOS is an ideal test for use in preschool asthma. Fractional exhaled nitric oxide (FeNO) levels correspond to eosinophilic inflammation and predict responsiveness to corticosteroids. Basic concepts of IOS, methodology, and interpretation, including available normative values, and recent findings regarding FeNO are reviewed in this article.

Asthma is a heterogeneous disorder described by a large number of clinical features. A growing body of literature on more specific asthma phenotypes provides evidence for a phenotype-based approach to management in which specific therapies are recommended based on patient and disease characteristics. This understanding, coupled with an increase in the number of available therapies for children with asthma, as well as emerging therapies and phenotypic markers, will allow for improved asthma management in the future.

Treatment nonadherence in young children with asthma involves multiple factors and should be viewed within an ecological framework. Few interventions have targeted multiple bidirectional factors, however, and little research has examined which interventions may be most appropriate for young children. Additional research is needed to identify essential intervention components, and to determine how to sustain such interventions in at-risk communities. Pediatric psychologists, with training in psychosocial intervention, screening, and primary prevention models, may be uniquely equipped to partner with communities and medical settings to develop and sustain targeted interventions for young children with asthma.

Severe asthma is broadly defined as asthma requiring a high level of therapy, usually high doses of inhaled corticosteroids, to bring under control. Children who remain symptomatic despite such treatment are a heterogeneous population, and bear a high burden of disease and require high resource utilization. Children with severe asthma require a comprehensive evaluation, careful consideration of alternative diagnoses and comorbid conditions, assessment of medication adherence and environmental conditions, and frequent disease monitoring.

The inner-city is a well-established and well-studied location that includes children at high risk for high asthma prevalence and morbidity. A number of intrinsic and extrinsic risk factors contribute to asthma in inner-city populations. This review seeks to explore these risk factors and evaluate how they contribute to increased asthma morbidity. Previous literature has identified risk factors such as race and ethnicity, prematurity, obesity, and exposure to aeroallergens and pollutants. Environmental and medical interventions aimed at individual risk factors and specific asthma phenotypes have contributed to improved outcomes in the inner-city children with asthma.

Children with asthma experience frequent exacerbations that require careful care coordination among families, clinicians, and schools. Prior studies have shown that children with asthma miss more school each year compared with their healthy peers due to uncontrolled asthma symptoms. Successful school-based asthma programs have built strong partnerships among patients, their families, and clinicians to improve communication and the dissemination of asthma action plans and medications to schools. The widely endorsed School-based Asthma Management Program, consisting of 4 components, provides a comprehensive and expert-supported framework to coordinate care with schools.

Childhood asthma affects many children placing them at significant risk for health care utilization and school absences. Several new developments relevant to the field of pediatric asthma have occurred over the last 5 years; yet, there is much more to learn. It is poorly understood how to prevent the disease, optimally address environmental challenges, or effectively manage poor adherence. Moreover, it is not clear how to customize therapy by asthma phenotype, age group, high risk groups, or severity of disease. Highlights of advances in pediatric asthma are reviewed and multiple essential areas for further exploration and research are discussed.

IMMUNOLOGY AND ALLERGY CLINICS OF NORTH AMERICA

SERIES OF RELATED INTEREST

Pediatric Clinics of North America
Available at: https://www.pediatric.theclinics.com/

THE CLINICS ARE AVAILABLE ONLINE!
Access your subscription at:
www.theclinics.com

Foreword
Childhood Asthma
Recent Progress with Management and New Hope for Prevention

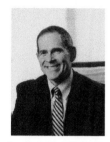

Stephen A. Tilles, MD
Consulting Editor

We began appreciating the existence of a pediatric asthma epidemic more than 2 decades ago, and in the years since then, the available treatment alternatives and paradigms have changed dramatically, including impressive improvements in symptom and objective testing outcomes in clinical studies, and an overall stabilization of prevalence and exacerbation rates.[1] However, pediatric asthma continues to be an important public health problem, and the overall disease burden shows no objective signs of shrinking in the near term. Fortunately, we may be headed for dramatic and impactful changes in the future. Recent insights into the importance of the interactions between early life bacterial exposures, viral infections, exposure to passive smoke and other pollutants, and aeroallergen sensitization have led to novel approaches to intervention with the goal of disease modification and/or prevention of asthma.

In this issue of *Immunology and Allergy Clinics of North America*, Drs Guilbert and Bacharier have assembled an internationally prominent group of authors to address cutting-edge topics relevant to the pathophysiology, diagnosis, management, and prevention of pediatric asthma. The issue tackles an incredibly complicated topic, yet is both thorough and practical, and will therefore serve as an invaluable reference for

Dr Tilles' consultant work for this issue of *Immunology and Allergy Clinics of North America* was completed before he became an employee of Aimmune Therapeutics.

Immunol Allergy Clin N Am 39 (2019) xiii–xiv
https://doi.org/10.1016/j.iac.2019.02.002
0889-8561/19/© 2019 Published by Elsevier Inc.

practicing allergists, pulmonologists, pediatricians, family physicians, and other health care providers who see children with asthma.

Stephen A. Tilles, MD
Aimmune Therapeutics
University of Washington
2410 Aurora Avenue N, #110
Seattle, WA 98105, USA

E-mail address:
Stephentilles@gmail.com

REFERENCE

1. Zahran HS, Bailey CM, Damon SA, et al. Vital signs: asthma in children–United States, 2001–2016. MMWR Morb Mortal Wkly Rep 2018;67(5):149–55.

Preface

Key Issues in Pediatric Asthma

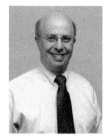 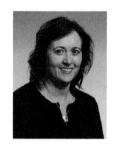

Leonard B. Bacharier, MD   Theresa W. Guilbert, MD, MS

Editors

Childhood asthma is characterized by airway inflammation, hyperresponsiveness, and variable airflow obstruction. It is a common disease that affects an estimated 6.8 million children in the United States,[1] which places them at significant risk for hospitalizations, emergency room visits, and school absences.[2-4] Asthma accounts for 13.8 million days of school missed annually and results in a significant social and economic burden for both families and the health care system.[1,2] Asthma also exerts a particularly heavy burden on children from racial and ethnic minorities, particularly those living in inner cities.[3,4] Management of pediatric asthma is challenging because disease phenotypes are heterogeneous and evolving. Often limited evidence is available to make therapeutic decisions, particularly in younger children, and is often extrapolated from adolescent and adult clinical trials. Asthma management encompasses treatment of the disease itself and management of comorbidities as well as patient and family education.

New concepts have emerged in the last decade regarding the risk factors, diagnosis, progression, and management of asthma and asthmalike symptoms during childhood. This issue focuses on the most recent developments, evidence, and novel ideas relevant to pediatric asthma. Key topic areas for recurrent wheezing and asthma in childhood include the risk factors for inception and progress of the disease, primary and secondary prevention, recent diagnostic techniques, management of preschool and school-aged children, treatment of severe asthma, personalization of treatment, and environmental exposures. New advances in self-management skill training and adherence monitoring and strategies to extend our pediatric asthma care beyond the traditional clinic and hospital settings are also discussed in this issue. Finally, we end the

Immunol Allergy Clin N Am 39 (2019) xv–xvi
https://doi.org/10.1016/j.iac.2019.02.001
0889-8561/19/© 2019 Published by Elsevier Inc.

immunology.theclinics.com

issue with highlights on future directions, which are important to advance our understanding of childhood asthma.

Leonard B. Bacharier, MD
Department of Pediatrics
Washington University School of Medicine
Campus Box 8116
660 South Euclid Avenue
St. Louis, MO 63110, USA

Theresa W. Guilbert, MD, MS
Department of Pediatrics
University of Cincinnati
Pulmonary Division
Cincinnati Children's Hospital
Medical Center
3333 Burnet Avenue
MLC 7049
Cincinnati, OH 45229, USA

E-mail addresses:
Bacharier_l@wustl.edu (L.B. Bacharier)
Theresa.Guilbert@cchmc.org (T.W. Guilbert)

REFERENCES

1. Zahran HS, Bailey CM, Damon SA, et al. Vital signs: asthma in children—United States, 2001–2016. MMWR Morb Mortal Wkly Rep 2018;67(5):149–55.
2. Nurmagambetov T, Kuwahara R, Garbe P. The economic burden of asthma in the United States, 2008-2013. Ann Am Thorac Soc 2018;15(3):348–56.
3. Weiss KB, Gergen PJ, Crain EF. Inner-city asthma. The epidemiology of an emerging US public health concern. Chest 1992;101(suppl 6):362S–7S.
4. Togias A, Fenton MJ, Gergen PJ, et al. Asthma in the inner city: the perspective of the National Institute of Allergy and Infectious Diseases. J Allergy Clin Immunol 2010;125(3):540–4.

Childhood Asthma Inception and Progression

Role of Microbial Exposures, Susceptibility to Viruses and Early Allergic Sensitization

Fernando D. Martinez, MD

KEYWORDS

- Asthma • Allergy • Rhinovirus • Prevention • Microbiome • Genetics

KEY POINTS

- Inappropriate responses to respiratory viruses, especially rhinovirus, and early allergic sensitization are the strongest contributors to the inception and persistence of early onset asthma.
- Children with genetically mediated alterations of immune regulatory mechanisms and who are insufficiently exposed to environmental microbes may be at the highest risk for early onset asthma.
- Mucosal colonization is not a passive process, but involves active interfaces between bacteria and the local immune system.

New concepts have emerged in the last decade regarding the incidence, risk factors, and progression of asthma and asthma-like symptoms during childhood. These issues have been addressed in dozens of longitudinally followed cohorts, and their results have considerably enriched the understanding of childhood asthma. The goal of this article is to focus on the most recent developments and novel ideas, especially those that point to new strategies for the primary and secondary prevention of the disease.

INCIDENCE OF CHILDHOOD ASTHMA

Many of the birth cohorts from which information on asthma incidence could be derived were enriched for children with a family history of asthma and allergies. It is fair to surmise that these studies would bias findings of the age distribution of asthma onset toward an earlier age. Long-term follow-up data from longitudinal studies may

Disclosure statement: The author was funded by grant HL132523 from the US National Heart, Lung, and Blood Institute.
Asthma and Airway Disease Research Center, The University of Arizona, 1501 North Campbell, Room 2350, Tucson, AZ 85724, USA
E-mail address: fdmartin@email.arizona.edu

also be biased by preferential retention of participants at increased risk for the disease. The most reliable information comes from large population samples in which assessment of incidence was based on use of asthma medication or other health care utilization-based indices. The National Asthma Program undertaken in Finland from 1994 to 2004 provided the most recent comprehensive data.[1] Its results indicate that asthma can start at any age, but the highest incidence occurs during the first 4 years of life, with a steady decrease thereafter, at least until the sixth decade of life. These findings confirmed older information from Rochester, Minnesota,[2] and particularly from the 1958 British Birth Cohort,[3] which followed 7000 persons born in England, Scotland, and Wales in a single week in 1958. It is thus unlikely that the marked peak in asthma incidence during the first years of life observed in the Finnish data may be caused by the influence of a significant number of transient wheezers,[4] whose symptoms will remit before they reach the school years.

The fact that new symptoms of asthma can start at any time during the lifetime and that inception most often occurs in early life suggests 2 major conclusions. On the 1 hand, the disease is fundamentally heterogeneous, and the umbrella of asthma may shelter many distinct illnesses starting at different ages, and all characterized by recurrent airway obstruction. On the other hand, the most frequent expression of the disease, early onset asthma, must be caused or triggered by factors that are active early postnatally or even intrauterine.

GENETICS OF EARLY ONSET ASTHMA

The results of 2 recent genome-wide association studies (GWAS) have provided strong support for the contention that early onset asthma may be a specific asthma phenotype, in which interactions between asthma loci and both viral respiratory illnesses and microbial exposures play a major role. By far the largest and most recent of these GWAS comprised more than 20,000 cases and over 100,000 controls from a multiancestry sample collected in a large number of countries.[5] This study confirmed that many loci distributed in the genome show strong association with asthma. The definition of asthma was based on physician diagnosis or standardized questionnaires, and it thus most likely included many of the different subillnesses that the diagnosis is likely to comprise. The study suggested that asthma is a polygenic disease, because it was powered to detect small signals and still, could only explain a small fraction of the total genetic variance of the disease. As suggested by a previous, smaller GWAS,[6] most loci identified were close to genes not known to be related to modulation of immunoglobulin E (IgE)- or Th2-mediated responses. By far the strongest signal detected was located at and around chromosome 17q21, a locus that has been consistently replicated in most of the largest asthma GWAS published to date. Of particular importance was the fact that Demenais and colleagues[5] identified 2 separate subloci within this single 17q locus: one near the *ORMDL3* gene and a second close to the *PGAP3* gene. Of note, the first of these signals was more strongly associated with childhood asthma, whereas the signal closer to *PGAP3* was stronger among adults. This finding thus replicated previous reports showing that the *ORMDL3* locus identifies a form of asthma that starts in early life.

A second asthma-related locus identified by GWAS,[7] but not replicated by Demenais and colleagues, was described in the *CDHR3* gene. The fact that a specific phenotype, namely, development of severe wheezing illnesses during the preschool years, was used in this study may explain the mismatch between the 2 GWAS results. Of importance, however, was the fact that recent functional studies demonstrated that CDHR3 is a major component of the receptor system for rhinovirus type C,[8] an important etiologic factor for asthma exacerbations, especially in young children. Moreover, the *CDHR3* at-risk allele was found to specifically alter in vitro responses to rhinovirus C,[8] suggesting a mechanism through which the genetic variant could increase the risk for severe wheezing illnesses.[9]

RHINOVIRUSES AND THE INCEPTION OF EARLY ONSET ASTHMA

The finding that a protein involved in the response to human rhinoviruses (HRV) could be a component of the genetics of early onset asthma supported the contention that HRV could play a significant role inception of the disease. Birth cohort studies in Madison, Wisconsin, and Perth, Australia,[10,11] had shown that children in whom HRV was isolated from the upper airway during wheezing illnesses early were more likely to develop early onset asthma by the age of 6 years than those who did not have HRV-related wheezing. Moreover, in the Madison cohort, children who had HRV-related wheezing illnesses in early life showed significant delays in lung function growth by the school years.[12] It remained unclear, however, what caused this increased susceptibility to HRV, and in which way it was connected to the subsequent development of early onset asthma.

Important new insights came from combining genetic and virologic data from the 2 separate birth cohorts. Caliskan and colleagues[13] studied the Madison birth cohort and a second one from Copenhagen and reported that the children with the highest risk for early onset asthma were those who had HRV-related wheezing illnesses in early life and were carriers of the at-risk allele in the *ORMDL3* locus. These findings suggested the possibility that this locus could explain at least in part the connection between early HRV illnesses and subsequent early onset asthma. The biologic mechanism explaining the HRV-ORMDL3 interaction remains unexplained, but insights come from studies of the *ORMDL3* locus in animal farming communities.

ANIMAL FARMING AND EARLY ONSET ASTHMA

For decades, the predominant paradigm explaining early onset asthma causation postulated that excessive exposures to allergens strongly associated with early onset asthma such as house dust mites were the main etiologic factors for the disease.[14] This idea inspired a handful of primary prevention trials,[15,16] comparing incidence of early onset asthma in children raised from birth in homes extensively treated to decrease exposure to mites with respect to those raised in control homes. These trials yielded mostly negative findings. These results were perplexing, because early sensitization to aeroallergens, and especially to house dust mites in many locales, is one of the strongest risk factors for the development of early onset asthma.[17]

The subsequent finding that children raised from birth on animal farms in the Alpine region were protected against the development of early onset asthma and early allergic sensitization[18] revolutionized understanding of the factors that determine the inception of the disease. A large cross-sectional study of children living in several countries across Europe confirmed this finding,[19] and suggested that environmental microbial burden could explain the protection, because a major correlate of the association between early onset asthma and animal farming was exposure to environmental bacteria and fungi.[20] It was also shown that children raised on an animal farm had decreased incidence of both transient wheezing and persistent, atopic wheezing as compared with those not exposed to farm animals.[19] Moreover, the trans-European study replicated in a completely different context the finding by Caliskan and colleagues[13] of an interaction between early wheezing illnesses and at-risk variants in the *ORMDL3* locus as determinants of early onset asthma in the early school years.[21] Of greater importance, however, was the fact that the same 17q alleles that conferred asthma risk in children with wheezing illnesses in early life granted strong protection against early onset asthma in children raised on animal farms.[21]

When combined, these findings contribute to the understanding of the role of the *ORMDL3* locus in the inception of early onset asthma. This locus comprises many genetic variants, which, in populations of European ancestry, are in high linkage disequilibrium (ie, travel together within parental chromosomes to their offspring) within an extensive genomic region of chromosome 17q21. The risk alleles for early onset asthma are present in approximately half of all chromosomes in populations of European origins, suggesting that unidentified, protective factors must have balanced during evolution the negative effects of an increased risk for early onset asthma. The fact that among children raised on animal farms the early onset asthma risk alleles at the ORMDL3 locus are associated with protection against the development of early onset asthma strongly suggests that a major mechanism that explains the decreased incidence of asthma in these children is protection against potential ill effects of viral respiratory infection in early life. The hypothesis emerging from these data is that, in the absence of high levels of microbial exposure in early life, *ORMDL3* enhances the clinical expression and the disruption of airway architecture associated with viral infection in early life. On the contrary, in the presence of microbial exposure, carriers of the *ORMDL3* risk alleles are protected against these ill effects. Because this hypothesis is based on still limited data, further functional and mechanistic studies are needed to confirm it.

HUMAN MICROBIOME AND THE INCEPTION OF EARLY ONSET ASTHMA

In parallel to studies of the environmental microbiome, assessment of the microbial content of both the upper airway and the stools in early life has provided new insights into the role of mucosae and microbes in determining asthma risk. Data from the Copenhagen birth cohort first showed that infants carrying 3 major pathogenic bacteria in their nasopharynx (ie, *Streptococcus pneumoniae, Moraxella catharralis*, and *Haemophilus influenzae*) were more likely to develop asthma by the age of 6 years than those not carrying these microbes.[22] In a more comprehensive analysis of the full microbiome, Teo and colleagues[23] confirmed that presence of these 3 species conferred increased risk for the subsequent development of asthma. These studies left unclear, however, if these bacterial pathogens could somehow trigger the mechanisms that lead to the inception of asthma or vice versa if their ability to colonize the upper airway of young infants at risk for asthma is a marker of alterations in the host's immune response at the mucosal level.[24] Of interest, Jartti and colleagues[25] studied 52 children aged 3 years or younger who were hospitalized with their first episode of severe wheezing and reported that 60% had a positive nasopharyngeal culture for at least 1 of the 3 previously mentioned pathogens. In a different study, isolation of these same microbes was associated with a similar risk of having wheezing episodes as the isolation of respiratory viruses from the upper airways of preschool children.[26] These results suggested that bacteria may be as likely as viruses to trigger episodes of airway obstruction, but still did not help clarify the causative role of bacteria in the inception of early onset asthma.

Cogent new data have emerged from studies of the fecal microbiome of young children who would go on to develop asthma or asthma-related phenotypes in the first years of life. Arrieta and colleagues[27] first showed that infants whose stools contained 4 species of bacteria (*Faecalibacterium, Lachnospira, Veillonella,* and *Rothia*) during the first months of life, but not at age 1, were protected against the development of atopic wheeze by the end of the first year of life. These same species, when administered orally to germ-free mice, who transmitted them to their offspring, protected the offspring against the development of allergic inflammation and bronchial hyperreactivity after sensitization with ovalbumin.[27] In a subsequent comprehensive assessment of the fecal microbiome during the first months of life, Fujimura and colleagues[28] identified 3 different microbial community patterns, dubbed NGM1, NGM2, and NGM3. Carriers of the NGM3 pattern, which showed lower relative abundance of certain bacteria (eg, *Bifidobacterium, Akkermansia,* and *Faecalibacterium*), were significantly more likely to develop physician-diagnosed asthma by age 4 years and allergic sensitization by age 2 years than carriers of the NGM1 pattern. The NGM3 pattern also showed a distinct fecal metabolome, enriched for proinflammatory metabolites. Taken together, these results suggest that the type of microbial communities that colonize the intestine during early infancy may influence immune responses in a distal organ such as the airway. This may occur either through direct effects of their metabolic products on somatic function or through the activation of protective immune mechanisms mediated through the intestinal mucosa. Support for the latter mechanism was provided by experiments using lyophilized bacterial products used empirically to prevent respiratory infections. Navarro and colleagues[29] showed that oral administration of these products blocked eosinophilic responses and the development bronchial hyperreactivity in mice sensitized and re-exposed to aeroallergens. They also showed that the lyophilizates interacted with dendritic cells in the gut mucosa, which in turn activated T-regulatory cells that migrated to the airway mucosa and were responsible for the protective effects attributable to the medicines.

Why bacteria that confer risk or protection against early onset asthma are able to colonize the airways and gut of different children is unknown. Because mucosal colonization is not a passive process but involves active interfaces between bacteria and the local immune system, it is likely that 3 factors are at play: genetic background of the individual, degree of maturation of the local immune response, and the timing of the exposure to microbes and their products during the first months of life. A cogent hypothesis, still to be tested, is that inadequate exposure to protective bacteria because of environmental sterilization and excessive antibiotic use may delay the development of the normal microbial-mucosal interface[30] and allow colonization of the airway and gut by pathogenic and asthma-inducing bacteria.

PROGRESSION OF EARLY ONSET ASTHMA INTO CHRONIC DISEASE: THE ROLE OF AEROALLERGEN SENSITIZATION

Longitudinal studies have shown that not all subjects who develop early onset asthma will go on to have symptoms that persist during the school years and into adult life. Stein and colleagues[31] showed that children who wheezed at age 6 and were sensitized to aeroallergens, and especially to the mold *Alternaria* in Tucson's desert environment, were much more likely to have persistent asthma at age 11 than nonatopic wheezers. Of interest, the diameter of the wheal elicited by the *Alternaria* antigen in the skin strongly correlated with the number of aeroallergens to which the child was sensitized,[32] suggesting that sensitivity to *Alternaria* was a marker for a global increased propensity to develop IgE responses to environmental stimuli. This hypothesis was supported by studies among children enrolled in the Dunedin cohort,[33] in which sensitization to house dust mites predicted which 9-year-old children would go on to have wheezing that persisted into adult life. Extending these findings, Illi and colleagues[34] reported that in the MAAS birth cohort in Germany, sensitization and exposure to perennial aeroallergens (house dust mites, dogs, and cats) during the first 3 years of life was strongly associated with the likelihood of having asthma that persisted beyond the early school years. They also showed that children who wheezed and were sensitized to perennial aeroallergens had significantly lower forced expiratory volume in 1 second (FEV_1)/forced vital capacity (FVC) ratio than those who were not sensitized. These results suggest that in early onset asthma, after the first hit associated with inappropriate responses to viruses, a second hit, aeroallergen sensitization, may be necessary to trigger airway remodeling and chronic airflow limitation, the hallmarks of persistent early onset asthma. This conclusion is supported by the finding that early allergic sensitization[35,36] (ie, during the first 3 years of life) is much more strongly associated with early onset asthma than late allergic sensitization.

The fact that the type of aeroallergen most strongly associated with this second hit differs so markedly by locale (eg, house dust mites in more humid areas, *Alternaria* in dry deserts) strongly suggests that it is not any specific allergen but, more likely, a general propensity to become sensitized to locally dominant aeroallergens that is responsible for the second hit. Moreover, in the Manchester, UK birth cohort, the factor most strongly associated with severe early onset asthma was early sensitization to multiple aeroallergens.[35]

The molecular mechanisms that determine the tendency to develop multiple early allergic sensitization and associated early onset asthma are the matter of intense research. Custovic and colleagues[37] recently assessed multiple cytokine responses by peripheral blood mononuclear cells (PBMCs) to HRV stimulation in over 300 11-year-old children enrolled in the Manchester birth cohort. They used machine-learning technologies and identified 6 cytokine response clusters. Children from 1 cluster, which had the lowest interferon induction and high induction of proinflammatory cytokines, showed all the characteristics associated with early onset asthma. Indeed, they were significantly more likely to be sensitized to aeroallergens by age 1 year, to have bronchiolitis in early life, to have persistent asthma symptoms up to age 16, and to have more severe symptoms between birth and adolescence.[37] This observation suggests the possibility that the susceptibility to respiratory viruses described earlier for early onset asthma and the tendency to develop early allergic sensitization may be mechanistically linked or have common origins. An objection to these observations in the Manchester cohort could be, however, that responses to HRV were assessed at age 11 and not in early life and therefore, that asthma and allergic sensitization may cause the subsequent patterns of HRV response. Against this latter interpretation is the observation from the Tucson birth cohort that diminished interferon gamma responses by PBMC to mitogenic stimuli at age 9 months were associated with increased subsequent risk for allergic sensitization to *Alternaria*[38] and for wheezing persisting up to 11 years of age.[39] Moreover, Bosco and colleagues[40] showed that school-aged children with more severe asthma (ie, associated with chronic airflow limitation) had diminished expression of interferon genes in sputum obtained during acute exacerbations compared with asthmatic children who had normal baseline lung function. Similarly, Johnston and colleagues have published several studies showing diminished interferon responses by bronchial epithelial cells in subjects with severe adult asthma.[41] Recent studies with ORMDL3-deficient mice further highlight the intertwined nature of the respiratory virus/allergic sensitization complex.[42] These mice were unable to mount an airway allergic response to *Alternaria*, the main aeroallergen associated with asthma in the desert Southwest. These animals showed no bronchial hyper-responsiveness or eosinophilia in response to *Alternaria*, but restoration of ORMDL3 expression using and adeno-associated virus vector fully reinstated these responses to the allergen. Thus, although ORMDL3 does not increase the risk of allergic sensitization,[43] it may increase susceptibility to an inflammatory response against aeroallergens in the airways.

Taken together, these results suggest the hypothesis that children with genetically mediated alterations of immune regulatory mechanisms that affect responses to both respiratory viruses and to aeroallergens and who are not exposed to protective mechanisms such as early microbial exposures may be at the highest risk of developing the most severe and persistent early onset asthma phenotypes.

The existence of a potential common mechanism for the development of early allergic sensitization and susceptibility to viral respiratory infection may also help resolve the question as to which of these 2 risk factors comes first.[44] Complex statistical assessments using data from the Madison birth cohort suggested that allergic sensitization precedes wheezing caused by HRV in early life.[45] The investigators argued that this sequential relationship supported a causal role for allergic sensitization, which would increase susceptibility to viruses and, by this mechanism, determine the inception of asthma. This interpretation, however, is not compatible with the finding that HRV interacts with the ORMDL3/17q locus to determine asthma susceptibility and that this interaction is independent of allergic sensitization.[13] In fact, several studies have failed to find any association between this locus and allergic sensitization.[43] It is important to stress that the Madison cohort was enriched for children with a family history of allergies. If a common pathogenic mechanism determines at least in part both early allergic sensitization and susceptibility to HRV, it is plausible to surmise that the timing of the expression of these 2 phenotypes may depend of the genetic background of the individual. Therefore, in children with a family history of allergies, skin test reactivity may come before HRV wheezing, and the opposite may be true in those without such family history,[23] without any implication as to which is the cause of the other.

SUMMARY

Strong epidemiologic observations from birth cohorts suggest that both inappropriate responses to respiratory viruses, especially HRV, and early allergic sensitization are the strongest contributors to the inception and persistence of early onset asthma. The most highly replicated GWAS hit for asthma is the so-called *ORMDL3* locus in chromosome 17q, and this locus seems to exert its effects by increasing susceptibility to HRV in early life. However, being raised on animal farms, which is highly protective against the development of asthma, blocks the increased susceptibility to early onset asthma associated with the ORMDL3 locus and decreases the incidence of both atopic and nonatopic wheezing in early life. Most available evidence indicates that the protective effect of animal farms is mediated by exposure to microbes, and this has suggested the prospect that pharmaceutical products containing protective bacteria could prevent early onset asthma. A primary wheezing lower respiratory tract illness prevention study using bacterial lyophilisates in high-risk infants and young children is already under way (trial number: NCT02148796). In addition to susceptibility to respiratory viruses, early sensitization to multiple aeroallergens appears to be essential for persistence of asthma beyond the preschool years and into adult life. A secondary prevention trial will soon test the hypothesis that anti-IgE therapy might decrease the risk for subsequent persistent asthma in aeroallergen-sensitized children with early onset asthma (trial number: NCT02570984).

REFERENCES

1. Haahtela T, Tuomisto LE, Pietinalho A, et al. A 10 year asthma programme in Finland: major change for the better. Thorax 2006;61:663–70.

2. Yunginger JW, Reed CE, O'Connell EJ, et al. A community-based study of the epidemiology of asthma. Incidence rates, 1964-1983. Am Rev Respir Dis 1992; 146:888–94.
3. Strachan DP, Butland BK, Anderson HR. Incidence and prognosis of asthma and wheezing illness from early childhood to age 33 in a national British cohort. BMJ 1996;312:1195–9.
4. Martinez FD, Wright AL, Taussig LM, et al. Asthma and wheezing in the first six years of life. The Group Health Medical Associates. N Engl J Med 1995;332: 133–8.
5. Demenais F, Margaritte-Jeannin P, Barnes KC, et al. Multiancestry association study identifies new asthma risk loci that colocalize with immune-cell enhancer marks. Nat Genet 2018;50:42–53.
6. Moffatt MF, Gut IG, Demenais F, et al. A large-scale, consortium-based genome-wide association study of asthma. N Engl J Med 2010;363:1211–21.
7. Bonnelykke K, Sleiman P, Nielsen K, et al. A genome-wide association study identifies CDHR3 as a susceptibility locus for early childhood asthma with severe exacerbations. Nat Genet 2014;46:51–5.
8. Bochkov YA, Watters K, Ashraf S, et al. Cadherin-related family member 3, a childhood asthma susceptibility gene product, mediates rhinovirus C binding and replication. Proc Natl Acad Sci U S A 2015;112:5485–90.
9. Bonnelykke K, Coleman AT, Evans MD, et al. CDHR3 genetics and rhinovirus C respiratory illnesses. Am J Respir Crit Care Med 2017;197(5):589–94.
10. Lemanske RF Jr, Jackson DJ, Gangnon RE, et al. Rhinovirus illnesses during infancy predict subsequent childhood wheezing. J Allergy Clin Immunol 2005;116: 571–7.
11. Kusel MM, de Klerk NH, Kebadze T, et al. Early-life respiratory viral infections, atopic sensitization, and risk of subsequent development of persistent asthma. J Allergy Clin Immunol 2007;119:1105–10.
12. Guilbert TW, Singh AM, Danov Z, et al. Decreased lung function after preschool wheezing rhinovirus illnesses in children at risk to develop asthma. J Allergy Clin Immunol 2011;128:532–8.e1-10.
13. Caliskan M, Bochkov YA, Kreiner-Moller E, et al. Rhinovirus wheezing illness and genetic risk of childhood-onset asthma. N Engl J Med 2013;368:1398–407.
14. Sporik R, Chapman MD, Platts-Mills TA. House dust mite exposure as a cause of asthma. Clin Exp Allergy 1992;22:897–906.
15. Custovic A, Simpson BM, Murray CS, et al. The National Asthma Campaign Manchester Asthma and Allergy Study. Pediatr Allergy Immunol 2002;13(Suppl 15): 32–7.
16. Toelle BG, Ng KK, Crisafulli D, et al. Eight-year outcomes of the Childhood Asthma Prevention Study. J Allergy Clin Immunol 2010;126:388–9, 389.e1-3.
17. Li J, Wang H, Chen Y, et al. House dust mite sensitization is the main risk factor for the increase in prevalence of wheeze in 13- to 14-year-old schoolchildren in Guangzhou city, China. Clin Exp Allergy 2013;43:1171–9.
18. Riedler J, Braun-Fahrlander C, Eder W, et al. Exposure to farming in early life and development of asthma and allergy: a cross-sectional survey. Lancet 2001;358: 1129–33.
19. Fuchs O, Genuneit J, Latzin P, et al. Farming environments and childhood atopy, wheeze, lung function, and exhaled nitric oxide. J Allergy Clin Immunol 2012;130: 382–388 e6.
20. Ege MJ, Mayer M, Normand AC, et al. Exposure to environmental microorganisms and childhood asthma. N Engl J Med 2011;364:701–9.

21. Loss GJ, Depner M, Hose AJ, et al. The early development of wheeze. environmental determinants and genetic susceptibility at 17q21. Am J Respir Crit Care Med 2016;193:889–97.

22. Bisgaard H, Hermansen MN, Buchvald F, et al. Childhood asthma after bacterial colonization of the airway in neonates. N Engl J Med 2007;357:1487–95.

23. Teo SM, Mok D, Pham K, et al. The infant nasopharyngeal microbiome impacts severity of lower respiratory infection and risk of asthma development. Cell Host Microbe 2015;17:704–15.

24. Martinez FD, Guerra S. Early origins of asthma. Role of microbial dysbiosis and metabolic dysfunction. Am J Respir Crit Care Med 2018;197:573–9.

25. Jartti T, Kuneinen S, Lehtinen P, et al. Nasopharyngeal bacterial colonization during the first wheezing episode is associated with longer duration of hospitalization and higher risk of relapse in young children. Eur J Clin Microbiol Infect Dis 2011; 30:233–41.

26. Bisgaard H, Hermansen MN, Bonnelykke K, et al. Association of bacteria and viruses with wheezy episodes in young children: prospective birth cohort study. BMJ 2010;341:c4978.

27. Arrieta MC, Stiemsma LT, Dimitriu PA, et al. Early infancy microbial and metabolic alterations affect risk of childhood asthma. Sci Transl Med 2015;7:307ra152.

28. Fujimura KE, Sitarik AR, Havstad S, et al. Neonatal gut microbiota associates with childhood multisensitized atopy and T cell differentiation. Nat Med 2016;22: 1187–91.

29. Navarro S, Cossalter G, Chiavaroli C, et al. The oral administration of bacterial extracts prevents asthma via the recruitment of regulatory T cells to the airways. Mucosal Immunol 2011;4:53–65.

30. Martinez FD. The human microbiome. Early life determinant of health outcomes. Ann Am Thorac Soc 2014;11(Suppl 1):S7–12.

31. Stein RT, Holberg CJ, Morgan WJ, et al. Peak flow variability, methacholine responsiveness and atopy as markers for detecting different wheezing phenotypes in childhood. Thorax 1997;52:946–52.

32. Halonen M, Stern DA, Wright AL, et al. *Alternaria* as a major allergen for asthma in children raised in a desert environment. Am J Respir Crit Care Med 1997;155: 1356–61.

33. Sears MR, Greene JM, Willan AR, et al. A longitudinal, population-based, cohort study of childhood asthma followed to adulthood. N Engl J Med 2003;349: 1414–22.

34. Illi S, von Mutius E, Lau S, et al. Perennial allergen sensitisation early in life and chronic asthma in children: a birth cohort study. Lancet 2006;368:763–70.

35. Simpson A, Tan VY, Winn J, et al. Beyond atopy: multiple patterns of sensitization in relation to asthma in a birth cohort study. Am J Respir Crit Care Med 2010;181: 1200–6.

36. Gergen PJ, Togias A. Inner city asthma. Immunol Allergy Clin North Am 2015;35: 101–14.

37. Custovic A, Belgrave D, Lin L, et al. Cytokine responses to rhinovirus and development of asthma, allergic sensitization, and respiratory infections during childhood. Am J Respir Crit Care Med 2018;197:1265–74.

38. Martinez FD, Stern DA, Wright AL, et al. Association of interleukin-2 and interferon-gamma production by blood mononuclear cells in infancy with parental allergy skin tests and with subsequent development of atopy. J Allergy Clin Immunol 1995;96:652–60.

39. Stern DA, Guerra S, Halonen M, et al. Low IFN-gamma production in the first year of life as a predictor of wheeze during childhood. J Allergy Clin Immunol 2007; 120:835–41.

40. Bosco A, Ehteshami S, Stern DA, et al. Decreased activation of inflammatory networks during acute asthma exacerbations is associated with chronic airflow obstruction. Mucosal Immunol 2010;3:399–409.

41. Johnston SL. Innate immunity in the pathogenesis of virus-induced asthma exacerbations. Proc Am Thorac Soc 2007;4:267–70.

42. Loser S, Gregory LG, Zhang Y, et al. Pulmonary ORMDL3 is critical for induction of *Alternaria*-induced allergic airways disease. J Allergy Clin Immunol 2017;139: 1496–14507 e3.

43. Bisgaard H, Bonnelykke K, Sleiman PM, et al. Chromosome 17q21 gene variants are associated with asthma and exacerbations but not atopy in early childhood. Am J Respir Crit Care Med 2009;179:179–85.

44. Sly PD, Kusel M, Holt PG. Do early-life viral infections cause asthma? J Allergy Clin Immunol 2010;125:1202–5.

45. Jackson DJ, Evans MD, Gangnon RE, et al. Evidence for a causal relationship between allergic sensitization and rhinovirus wheezing in early life. Am J Respir Crit Care Med 2012;185:281–5.

Potential Strategies and Targets for the Prevention of Pediatric Asthma

Brooke I. Polk, MD*, Leonard B. Bacharier, MD

KEYWORDS

- Asthma • Prevention • Microbiome • Vitamin D

KEY POINTS

- Exposure to a diverse microbial environment is likely protective versus asthma development, with a "critical window" of opportunity to alter the host microbiome in early infancy.
- Fetal exposure to appropriate amounts of vitamin D or fish oil could prevent recurrent wheeze or asthma.
- Modification of the host response to allergens via allergen immunotherapy may help to prevent asthma, although the duration of the effect is unclear.
- Prevention of viral respiratory tract infections shows promise for asthma prevention.

INTRODUCTION

Asthma is the most common chronic disease of childhood, resulting in missed school days and significant social and economic burden for both families and the health care system.[1–3] Identification of potentially modifiable environmental and host risk factors for asthma development (**Fig. 1**) has allowed for the beginning of a paradigm shift from disease treatment toward primary asthma prevention, and studies are underway to determine how best to prevent the development of asthma in children. This article reviews the effect of environmental exposures, host factors, and treatment of viral illnesses on the evolution of childhood asthma; summarizes successful primary prevention strategies; and identifies future areas of need.

Disclosures: Dr B.I. Polk has no disclosures. Dr L.B. Bacharier reports grants from NIH; personal fees from GlaxoSmithKline, Genentech/Novartis, Merck, DBV Technologies, Teva, Boehringer Ingelheim, AstraZeneca, WebMD/Medscape, Sanofi/Regeneron, Vectura, and Circassia.
Edward Mallinckrodt Department of Pediatrics, Division of Allergy, Immunology, and Pulmonary Medicine, Washington University in St. Louis, One Children's Place, Campus Box 8116, St Louis, MO 63110-1077, USA
* Corresponding author.
E-mail address: bpolk@wustl.edu

Immunol Allergy Clin N Am 39 (2019) 151–162
https://doi.org/10.1016/j.iac.2018.12.010
0889-8561/19/© 2018 Elsevier Inc. All rights reserved.
immunology.theclinics.com

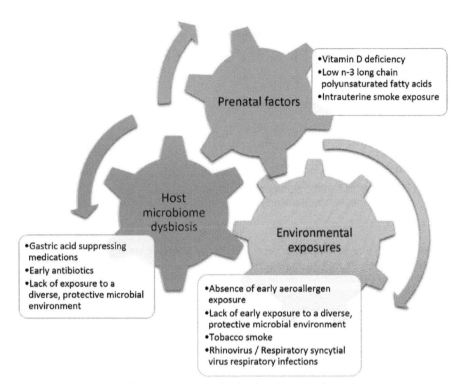

Fig. 1. Factors associated with an increased risk of asthma development.

MODIFIABLE ENVIRONMENTAL EXPOSURES: AEROALLERGENS AND ENVIRONMENTAL TOBACCO SMOKE

Multiple epidemiologic studies have demonstrated significant correlations between irritant and aeroallergen exposures, or lack thereof, and the subsequent development of recurrent wheeze or asthma in children.[4–6] Asthma prevalence is notably higher in developed countries, suggesting that the identification and alteration of modifiable environmental risk factors could decrease the risk of developing asthma. Although earlier studies yielded conflicting results regarding early aeroallergen exposure and asthma development, current data suggest that exposure to high levels of concomitant allergens and diverse environmental bacteria in the first year of life among high-risk children growing up in an urban environment is associated with reduced likelihoods of recurrent wheeze and asthma at ages 3 and 7 years.[4,7] Rural farming environments rich in microbes and aeroallergens also seem to be protective for asthma, allergic rhinitis (AR), and atopic sensitization.[8]

To evaluate the effects of the urban environment on asthma development, the Inner-City Asthma Consortium initiated the Urban Environment and Childhood Asthma study, an ongoing birth cohort assessing the factors associated with asthma development among inner-city children with at least 1 atopic parent.[9] Higher indoor levels of cockroach, mouse, and cat allergens during infancy were associated with a lower risk of asthma development at age 7 years,[4] suggesting that early indoor allergen avoidance is unlikely to be an effective strategy to reduce asthma prevalence, at least among inner-city children.

Environmental tobacco smoke exposure, including during the prenatal period, has been identified as another independent predictor of asthma development among the Urban Environment and Childhood Asthma cohort; children with higher levels of umbilical cord cotinine were at heightened risk of developing asthma.[4] A 2012 meta-analysis of 79 prospective studies concluded that prenatal or postnatal passive smoke exposure is associated with a 30% to 70% increased risk of incident wheeze in children (odds ratio, 1.7 in children aged $\leq$2 years; 95% confidence interval, 1.35–2.53) and a 21% to 85% increase in incident asthma (odds ratio, 1.85 in children aged $\leq$2 years; 95% confidence interval, 1.24–2.35).[5] Recently, a systematic review of 2 population-based birth cohorts demonstrated that smoke exposure at any age is associated with impaired lung function associated with persistent wheeze and asthma.[6] These results strongly suggest that interventions to decrease prenatal and postnatal smoke exposure may reduce asthma incidence and improve lung function in children.

HYGIENE HYPOTHESIS AND MICROBIOME DYSBIOSIS

The "hygiene" or "old friends" hypothesis postulates that decreased contact with microbial pathogens early in life leads to immune tolerance defects, resulting in heightened susceptibility to atopic disorders.[10] Early life exposures, including antibiotics, formula feeding, and gastric acid suppressive medications, may modify commensal intestinal microflora, causing dysbiosis and subsequent redirection toward a proallergic and proasthmatic T helper 2 phenotype.[11,12] Acid-suppressing medications decrease the digestion of proteins and may affect antigen processing. A recent cohort study of almost 800,000 children found positive associations between the use of gastric acid-reducing medications in the first 6 months of life and subsequent asthma (adjusted hazard ratio, 1.25 [95% confidence interval, 1.21–1.29] for H2 receptor blockers; adjusted hazard ratio, 1.41 [95% confidence interval, 1.31–1.52] for proton pump inhibitors). In the same study, antibiotic use in the first 6 months of life was associated with a 2-fold increased risk of childhood asthma (adjusted hazard ratio, 2.09; 95% confidence interval, 1.29–1.40).[11]

Increasing evidence supports a key association between respiratory and gastrointestinal microbiota and asthma, with notable differences in the microbiota between asthmatic and nonasthmatic individuals.[13,14]

Although previously thought to be relatively devoid of bacteria, sequencing of 16s ribosomal RNA has facilitated the discovery of a diverse microbial population within the human lower respiratory tract.[15] The respiratory microbiome changes throughout the first few years of life, reaching an adultlike composition around the age of 3, although neonates nasopharyngeally colonized with *Streptococcus pneumoniae, Haemophilus influenza*, and/or *Moraxella catarrhalis* at just 1 month of age are at 2 to 4 times greater risk for recurrent wheeze and asthma.[16,17] Examination of the lung microbiota of asthmatic patients consistently reveals more proteobacteria including *H influenzae, Pseudomonas, Neisseria*, and *Burkholderia* than in nonasthmatic individuals, independent of age, asthma severity, or treatment with corticosteroids.[13,18] Therapeutic strategies targeting the airway microbiome could be potentially valuable in asthma prevention, though this has not yet been pursued.

The influence of the gut microbiome on atopy development is an ongoing area of study, with evidence of a "critical window" in which intestinal dysbiosis perhaps irreversibly alters human immune development.[19] Perinatal antibiotic exposure is associated with higher serum IgE levels and fewer colon regulatory T cells in murine models,[20] and infants at risk of asthma have transient intestinal dysbiosis in the first 100 days of life that is not apparent at 1 year of age, suggesting that prenatal or neonatal intervention is crucial if modification of this dysbiotic state is targeted as an intervention to prevent asthma.[21] A study of 319 children enrolled in the Canadian Healthy Infant Longitudinal Development (CHILD) cohort found a significant reduction in the abundance of 4 genera—*Faecalibacterium, Lachnospira, Veillonella,* and *Rothia* (collectively termed FLVR)—in the stool of children who went on to develop atopic wheezing. Upon inoculation with FLVR, germ-free mice produced offspring with significantly reduced airway inflammation, implying a causal role of these 4 genera in protection from asthma.[21] Although there is no evidence to date for a protective effect of infant or maternal probiotic administration with either *Lactobacillus* or *Bifidobacterium* genera on the development of incident wheeze or lower respiratory tract infection (RTI) in infants,[22] perhaps supplementation with the FLVR genera could reduce the risk of asthma.

A striking example of the hygiene hypothesis is the farm effect, a well-studied phenomenon wherein children residing on farms have a significantly lower risk of recurrent wheeze and asthma, with a protective effect related to the diversity of microbial exposure.[17,23,24] To determine the effect of a traditional farming environment on immune response, a landmark 2016 study evaluated environmental exposures and immune profiles of children in distinct US Amish and Hutterite agricultural populations.[25] Despite similarities in lifestyle and genetic ancestry, Amish children have a strikingly lower prevalence of asthma and allergic sensitization relative to Hutterite children[26]; compared with Hutterites' large, industrialized farms, the Amish live on single dairy farms and use livestock for transportation. The authors found differences in microbial dust composition, significantly higher endotoxin levels in Amish house dust (6.8 times that of Hutterite homes), and profound disparities in innate immune cell phenotype and function between the 2 populations.[25] Interestingly, a subsequent analysis showed that, in a mouse model, inhalation of Hutterite barn dust can inhibit allergen-induced airway hyperresponsiveness and specific IgE. Overall, these findings suggest that Hutterite children perhaps lack early access to protective exposures, although specific protective microbes were not identified.

These findings may be generalizable to a larger and more diverse population, because aeroallergen concentration is directly correlated with differences in house dust microbiota in the Urban Environment and Childhood Asthma inner-city cohort discussed elsewhere in this article.[4,9] The homes of children who did not develop asthma more often contained *Kocuria,* an organism known to produce a macrolide with activity against *Staphylococcus* species, and *Bifidobacterium* and *Acinetobacter,* both of which protect against aeroallergen sensitization in mouse models.[27,28] In contrast, homes with a child who developed asthma were more likely to be enriched with the taxa *Staphylococcus, Haemophilus, Corynebacterium,* and *Sphingomonas.*[4] These disparities suggest that modification of environmental bacterial exposures in early life may influence the risk of asthma development, presumably through modification of the child's gastrointestinal and airway microbiomes.

EFFECTS OF MATERNAL DIET AND NUTRITIONAL SUPPLEMENTATION

Another factor is the westernized lifestyle, with increased time spent indoors and a diet dominated by processed, modified foods generally deficient in vitamins and minerals.[29] Increasing evidence points to the effect of the maternal diet on susceptibility to atopic disorders, raising the possibility that altering the prenatal diet is a potentially effective and inexpensive method of primary prevention for multiple inflammatory diseases.[30] The strongest data linking maternal dietary supplementation and asthma prevention exist for maternal vitamin D and fish oil, with limited data on folate.

Vitamin D has beneficial effects on innate and adaptive immunity, and maternal vitamin D is involved in fetal immune system development and lung maturation.[31,32] Vitamin D deficiency has long been proposed as a risk factor for asthma, and the recent increase in the prevalence of vitamin D deficiency mirrors the increase in asthma.[33] Higher maternal vitamin D intake is associated with reduced rates of recurrent wheeze in early childhood.[34,35]

Although a metaanalysis of 34 observational studies concluded that significant evidence does not exist to support an impact of vitamin D supplementation on asthma,[36] randomized controlled trials have yielded encouraging results. A study of 623 women from the Copenhagen Prospective Studies on Asthma (COPSAC$_{2010}$) cohort randomized women to receive either 2400 or 400 IU vitamin D from 24 weeks' gestation through delivery. Children born to mothers receiving the higher dose of vitamin D had nonsignificant but lower risk of persistent wheeze (hazard ratio, 0.76; 95% confidence interval, 0.52–1.12).[37] Similarly, the Vitamin D Antenatal Asthma Reduction Trial (VDAART) randomized 881 pregnant women at risk of having a child with asthma to either 4400 or 400 IU vitamin D daily starting at 10 to 18 weeks' gestation. The incidence of asthma or recurrent wheeze by age 3 years was 6.1% lower in children of women who received 4400 IU daily, although statistical significance was not attained ($P = .051$).[38] A follow-up study showed that children of mothers with an initial vitamin D level of greater than 30 ng/mL who were randomized to the intervention group had a significantly lower risk of asthma or recurrent wheeze by age 3 years (adjusted odds ratio, 0.42; 95% confidence interval, 0.19–0.91) compared with those with initial levels of less than 20 ng/mL randomized to placebo, suggesting that adequate vitamin D levels as early as in the first trimester (and potentially before conception), and maintained throughout pregnancy, may be necessary for asthma prevention.[39] This finding was replicated in combined analysis of the VDAART and COPSAC$_{2010}$ cohorts, with a risk reduction of almost 50% in offspring of mothers with initial vitamin D level of greater than 30 ng/mL who received supplementation.[40] Additional studies are necessary to further evaluate this question.

In 1997, Black and Sharpe[41] described an association between the increase in atopy with changes in dietary fat consumption in the Western diet, namely the increased use of plant-based oils containing omega-6-polyunsaturated fatty acids (n-6 PUFAs) such as linoleic acid, reduced use of animal fats (butter/lard), and decreased consumption of oily fish products containing n-3 long chain PUFAs (LCPUFAs). Because linoleic acid is a precursor to arachidonic acid, the increase in n-6 PUFA consumption can be linked to the production of prostaglandins including prostaglandin E2, which promotes T helper 2 cell differentiation. Dietary supplementation of asthmatic patients with n-3 LCPUFAs is ineffective,[42] but its use in preventing asthma has shown promise. Although a 2015 Cochrane review found little evidence to support maternal n-3 PUFA supplementation for reduction of allergic disease in children,[43] significant heterogeneity in included studies limited the findings; 2 recent large randomized controlled trials showed a benefit of prenatal fish oil supplementation on the prevention of wheeze in offspring.[44,45]

In 1 study, 736 women were randomized to receive either 2.4 g fish oil daily versus olive oil placebo starting at 24 weeks gestation, and 695 children were followed for 5 years. Children whose mothers received fish oil had a 30.7% overall reduced risk of persistent wheeze or asthma, with the greatest benefit seen in mothers with the lowest baseline LCPUFA levels before randomization (54.1%), with a number needed to treat of 6.[45] The second study examined adult offspring (aged 18–19 years) of mothers randomized to 2.7 g fish oil (vs olive oil vs no intervention) in the third trimester. Maternal fish oil supplementation was associated with a decreased probability of asthma medication prescription and an in-hospital discharge diagnosis of asthma in adult offspring.[44] These findings suggest a potentially beneficial effect of fish oil supplementation during pregnancy, although capsules are generally unpalatable and it may be challenging for some mothers to take multiple pills or to afford the financial cost of supplementation.[46] Of note, initial blood levels of n-3 LCPUFAs correlated with reported maternal fish ingestion; feasibly, targeting women with the least fish intake would be most advantageous, because the study doses of 2.4 to 2.7 g fish oil are roughly 20 times the normal daily n-3 LCPUFA intake in the United States.[45]

Prenatal folate exposure was formerly thought to be a risk factor for childhood atopy, owing to its ability to donate methyl groups and thereby epigenetically modify DNA.[47] Results of studies are mixed, and many studies do not include blood folate levels.[48,49] A recent prospective cohort study actually found a modest decrease in the odds of wheeze at age 3 among offspring of women high plasma folate levels in the second trimester (adjusted odds ratio, 0.67; 95% confidence interval, 0.46–0.97), although the finding was not replicated for third trimester folate levels.[50] These data certainly do not support a harmful effect of prenatal folate exposure on childhood atopic disease.

MODIFYING THE IMMUNE RESPONSE TO ALLERGENS

AR affects 2% to 25% of children, with steadily increasing prevalence.[51] Often preceding the development of asthma, AR is an independent risk factor for asthma development.[51,52] Although strict early avoidance of environmental allergens has generally not proven beneficial in the prevention of asthma in the general population,[53] evidence from small trials suggests that treatment of AR with allergen immunotherapy can prevent progression of AR to allergic asthma.[54–56] The first randomized trial designed to assess the efficacy of subcutaneous immunotherapy included 44 subjects with AR and bronchial hyperresponsiveness monosensitized to dust mite. After 2 years of subcutaneous immunotherapy, the methacholine provocative dose to elicit a 20% decrease in the Forced expiratory volume in 1 second increased 4-fold in the treatment group, and no treatment subjects developed asthma (vs 9% of placebo subjects).[57] Similar results were produced in children with AR sensitized to birch and/or grass pollen, with persistence of the preventative effect for at least 10 years.[58]

Asthma prevention results are not as robust for sublingual immunotherapy, although recently published results of the GRAZAX Asthma Prevention (GAP) study are somewhat encouraging. In 812 nonasthmatic children with AR sensitized to Timothy pollen, sublingual Timothy immunotherapy (GRAZAX, ALK-Abello, Denmark) given for 3 consecutive allergy seasons did not decrease incident asthma in 2-year follow-up, although asthma symptoms and medication use were reduced compared with placebo (odds ratio, 0.66; $P<.36$).[59]

Whereas a 2017 metaanalysis of 32 studies of allergen immunotherapy administered by any route found a short-term protective effect versus asthma (relative risk, 0.40; 95% confidence interval, 0.30–0.52), there was inconclusive evidence that benefit was maintained.[60] Well-conduced randomized controls with long-term outcomes are lacking.

Studies evaluating the effects of disruption in the atopic march, specifically in the prevention of atopic dermatitis and food allergy, have generally been precluded from examining asthma outcomes owing to short duration.[61] The PreventADALL multinational birth cohort (NCT02449850) seeks to determine if early, low-cost interventions could alter the course of atopic disease; infants are randomized to 1 of 4 groups, including observation only, early emollient use, early food introduction, and a combination of early interventions. Because these children will be studied through 2044, long-term outcomes, including effects on asthma prevention, will be possible. Also of note, a recent follow-up of the Learning Early About Peanut (LEAP) cohort noted that early consumption of peanut in high-risk infants is disease and allergen specific, and although reducing the risk of peanut allergy, this approach does not prevent the development of other atopic diseases, including asthma.[62]

ALTERING THE IMMUNE RESPONSE TO MICROBES

Viral RTIs are the most common cause of recurrent wheeze in infants, and wheezing illnesses in the context of infections with human rhinovirus and respiratory syncytial virus (RSV) are strong predictors of asthma development in children.[63,64] In 1 cohort, RSV bronchiolitis requiring hospitalization during infancy conferred a 50% likelihood of physician-diagnosed asthma by age 7 years, potentially mediated by the chemokine CCL5 (RANTES).[65] In the high risk for atopy Childhood Origins of ASThma (COAST) cohort, wheezing with human rhinovirus infection in the first year of life was associated with an increased risk of school-age asthma by 3-fold, and 90% of children with wheeze during human rhinovirus infection in the third year of life had developed asthma at age 6 years.[66]

Several therapies to decrease the incidence or severity of these RTIs have been evaluated, including prophylactic vaccination, antiinflammatory therapies, and immunostimulatory agents, under the premise that prevention or modulation of the acute illness will confer long-term protection from recurrent wheezing and asthma.

To identify a causal relationship between initial RSV infection and recurrent wheeze, the MAKI trial evaluated the effect of the anti-RSV monoclonal antibody palavizumab administration during RSV season in 429 otherwise healthy late preterm infants. Compared with placebo, palavizumab treatment reduced the number of wheezing days by 61% in the first year of life, even outside of RSV season, suggesting that primary prevention of RSV was an effective strategy in reducing all-cause wheezing.[67] After 6 years, this mode of RSV prevention was associated with decreased parent-reported wheeze but not in physician-diagnosed asthma or lung function.[68] Clinical trials of a maternal RSV vaccination (NCT02624947) and of an extended half-life anti-RSV monoclonal antibody (NCT 02878330) are underway. However, with an estimated direct cost of $10,665 for 5 monthly doses, it is not feasible to dose every infant with a full season of palavizumab therapy.[69]

Macrolide antibiotics have been proposed as a more cost-effective strategy, because these agents exhibit both antineutrophilic and antibacterial effects.[70] After azithromycin was shown to attenuate airway inflammation in a mouse model of viral bronchiolitis,[71] a pilot study of 40 infants hospitalized with RSV bronchiolitis randomized subjects to either 14 days of azithromycin versus placebo. Compared with placebo, azithromycin decreased upper airway IL-8 levels and resulted in decreased recurrent wheeze and fewer days with wheezing.[72] Interestingly, azithromycin modified the upper airway microbiome, with significantly decreased *Moraxella* abundance in the treatment group. Lower *Moraxella* abundance was independently associated with decreased odds of recurrent wheeze.[73] An ongoing trial (NCT02911935) aims to evaluate the effects of azithromycin on the upper airway microbiome and on recurrent wheeze during the preschool years.

Because most RTIs are viral, with hundreds of possible etiologies, vaccination for each individual virus is not a feasible prophylactic solution. Immunostimulatory agents enhance innate and adaptive immune response to infection by targeting the gut–lung immune axis.[74] Of the immunostimulatory agents, OM-85 BV (Broncho-Vaxom, OM Pharma, St. Gallen, Switzerland) is the most well-studied in RTI prevention. OM-85 BV is a bacterial lysate immunomodulator composed of 21 lyophilized strains of common respiratory pathogens, including *Haemophilus influenza*; *Streptococcus pneumoniae, pyogenes,* and *viridans*; *Klebsiella pneumoniae* and *ozaenae*; *Staphylococcus aureus*; and *M catarrhalis*, thought to exert efficacy by inhibiting T helper 2–mediated inflammation via gut dendritic cell activation and regulatory T-cell mobilization to the lung. Randomized controlled trials have demonstrated the efficacy of OM-85 BV in a reduction of the rate and duration of wheezing in children with recurrent RTIs.[74,75] A Cochrane analysis demonstrated a decrease in acute RTIs by 36%,[76] and an ongoing 36-month phase II trial is examining if OM-85 BV given regularly for 2 years to at-risk children ages 6 to 18 months of age (NCT02148796) decrease the likelihood of recurrent wheeze.

SUMMARY AND FUTURE CONSIDERATIONS

The increase in asthma prevalence necessitates the identification and alteration of modifiable risk factors to promote primary disease prevention. Evidence suggests that maternal diet modification resulting in fetal exposure to appropriate amounts of vitamin D or fish oil could prevent recurrent wheeze or asthma, and that early exposure to a diverse microbial environment is likely protective, with a likely critical window of opportunity to alter the host microbiome in very early infancy. Modification of the host response to allergens via specific allergen immunotherapy may prevent asthma, although the typical subcutaneous route of administration is time constraining. The prevention and modification of viral RTIs, a known risk factor for asthma, also shows promise and is under intense investigation. Immunostimulatory agents may also have a role in enhancing innate and adaptive immune response to infection by targeting the gut–lung immune axis. Ongoing trials and longitudinal birth cohort studies will help to identify additional protective strategies, because asthma prevention is clearly multifactorial.

REFERENCES

1. CDC - asthma - data and surveillance. Available at: http://www.cdc.gov/asthma/asthmadata.htm. Accessed June 1, 2018.

2. Vital signs: asthma in children - United States, 2001-2016. 2018. Available at: https://www.cdc.gov/mmwr/volumes/67/wr/mm6705e1.htm?s_cid=mm6705e1_w. Accessed June 1, 2018.

3. Nurmagambetov T, Kuwahara R, Garbe P. The economic burden of asthma in the United States, 2008-2013. Ann Am Thorac Soc 2018;15:348–56.

4. O'Connor GT, Lynch SV, Bloomberg GR, et al. Early-life home environment and risk of asthma among inner-city children. J Allergy Clin Immunol 2018;141: 1468–75.

5. Burke H, Leonardi-Bee J, Hashim A, et al. Prenatal and passive smoke exposure and incidence of asthma and wheeze: systematic review and meta-analysis. Pediatrics 2012;129:735–44.

6. Belgrave DCM, Granell R, Turner SW, et al. Lung function trajectories from preschool age to adulthood and their associations with early life factors: a retrospective analysis of three population-based birth cohort studies. Lancet Respir Med 2018;6(7):526–34.

7. Lynch SV, Wood RA, Boushey H, et al. Effects of early-life exposure to allergens and bacteria on recurrent wheeze and atopy in urban children. J Allergy Clin Immunol 2014;134:593–601.e12.
8. Riedler J, Braun-Fahrländer C, Eder W, et al. Exposure to farming in early life and development of asthma and allergy: a cross-sectional survey. Lancet 2001;358: 1129–33.
9. Gern JE, Visness CM, Gergen PJ, et al. The Urban Environment and Childhood Asthma (URECA) birth cohort study: design, methods, and study population. BMC Pulm Med 2009;9:17.
10. van Tilburg Bernardes E, Arrieta MC. Hygiene hypothesis in asthma development: is hygiene to blame? Arch Med Res 2017;48:717–26.
11. Mitre E, Susi A, Kropp LE, et al. Association between use of acid-suppressive medications and antibiotics during infancy and allergic diseases in early childhood. JAMA Pediatr 2018;172:e180315.
12. Larsen JM, Brix S, Thysen AH, et al. Children with asthma by school age display aberrant immune responses to pathogenic airway bacteria as infants. J Allergy Clin Immunol 2014;133:1008–13.
13. Huang YJ, Nelson CE, Brodie EL, et al. Airway microbiota and bronchial hyperresponsiveness in patients with suboptimally controlled asthma. J Allergy Clin Immunol 2011;127:372–81.e1-3.
14. Cardenas PA, Cooper PJ, Cox MJ, et al. Upper airways microbiota in antibiotic-naïve wheezing and healthy infants from the tropics of rural Ecuador. PLoS One 2012;7:e46803.
15. Hilty M, Burke C, Pedro H, et al. Disordered microbial communities in asthmatic airways. PLoS One 2010;5:e8578.
16. Bisgaard H, Hermansen MN, Buchvald F, et al. Childhood asthma after bacterial colonization of the airway in neonates. N Engl J Med 2007;357:1487–95.
17. Man WH, de Steenhuijsen Piters WA, Bogaert D. The microbiota of the respiratory tract: gatekeeper to respiratory health. Nat Rev Microbiol 2017;15:259–70.
18. von Mutius E. The microbial environment and its influence on asthma prevention in early life. J Allergy Clin Immunol 2016;137:680–9.
19. Cahenzli J, Köller Y, Wyss M, et al. Intestinal microbial diversity during early-life colonization shapes long-term IgE levels. Cell Host Microbe 2013;14:559–70.
20. Russell SL, Gold MJ, Willing BP, et al. Perinatal antibiotic treatment affects murine microbiota, immune responses and allergic asthma. Gut Microbes 2013;4: 158–64.
21. Arrieta MC, Stiemsma LT, Dimitriu PA, et al. Early infancy microbial and metabolic alterations affect risk of childhood asthma. Sci Transl Med 2015;7:307ra152.
22. Azad MB, Coneys JG, Kozyrskyj AL, et al. Probiotic supplementation during pregnancy or infancy for the prevention of asthma and wheeze: systematic review and meta-analysis. BMJ 2013;347:f6471.
23. Fuchs O, Genuneit J, Latzin P, et al. Farming environments and childhood atopy, wheeze, lung function, and exhaled nitric oxide. J Allergy Clin Immunol 2012;130: 382–8.e6.
24. Birzele LT, Depner M, Ege MJ, et al. Environmental and mucosal microbiota and their role in childhood asthma. Allergy 2017;72:109–19.
25. Stein MM, Hrusch CL, Gozdz J, et al. Innate immunity and asthma risk in Amish and Hutterite farm children. N Engl J Med 2016;375:411–21.
26. Ober C, Sperling AI, von Mutius E, et al. Immune development and environment: lessons from Amish and Hutterite children. Curr Opin Immunol 2017;48:51–60.

27. Feleszko W, Jaworska J, Rha RD, et al. Probiotic-induced suppression of allergic sensitization and airway inflammation is associated with an increase of T regulatory-dependent mechanisms in a murine model of asthma. Clin Exp Allergy 2007;37:498–505.

28. Debarry J, Hanuszkiewicz A, Stein K, et al. The allergy-protective properties of Acinetobacter lwoffii F78 are imparted by its lipopolysaccharide. Allergy 2010; 65:690–7.

29. Thomas D. A study on the mineral depletion of the foods available to us as a nation over the period 1940 to 1991. Nutr Health 2003;17:85–115.

30. Devereux G. The increase in the prevalence of asthma and allergy: food for thought. Nat Rev Immunol 2006;6:869–74.

31. Beard JA, Bearden A, Striker R. Vitamin D and the anti-viral state. J Clin Virol 2011;50:194–200.

32. Litonjua AA. Childhood asthma may be a consequence of vitamin D deficiency. Curr Opin Allergy Clin Immunol 2009;9:202–7.

33. Litonjua AA, Weiss ST. Is vitamin D deficiency to blame for the asthma epidemic? J Allergy Clin Immunol 2007;120:1031–5.

34. Camargo CA, Rifas-Shiman SL, Litonjua AA, et al. Maternal intake of vitamin D during pregnancy and risk of recurrent wheeze in children at 3 y of age. Am J Clin Nutr 2007;85:788–95.

35. Devereux G, Litonjua AA, Turner SW, et al. Maternal vitamin D intake during pregnancy and early childhood wheezing. Am J Clin Nutr 2007;85:853–9.

36. Pacheco-González RM, García-Marcos L, Morales E. Prenatal vitamin D status and respiratory and allergic outcomes in childhood: a meta-analysis of observational studies. Pediatr Allergy Immunol 2018;29:243–53.

37. Chawes BL, Bønnelykke K, Stokholm J, et al. Effect of vitamin D3 supplementation during pregnancy on risk of persistent wheeze in the offspring: a randomized clinical trial. JAMA 2016;315:353–61.

38. Litonjua AA, Carey VJ, Laranjo N, et al. Effect of prenatal supplementation with vitamin D on asthma or recurrent wheezing in offspring by age 3 years: the VDAART randomized clinical trial. JAMA 2016;315:362–70.

39. Wolsk HM, Harshfield BJ, Laranjo N, et al. Vitamin D supplementation in pregnancy, prenatal 25(OH)D levels, race, and subsequent asthma or recurrent wheeze in offspring: secondary analyses from the Vitamin D Antenatal Asthma Reduction Trial. J Allergy Clin Immunol 2017;140:1423–9.e5.

40. Wolsk HM, Chawes BL, Litonjua AA, et al. Prenatal vitamin D supplementation reduces risk of asthma/recurrent wheeze in early childhood: a combined analysis of two randomized controlled trials. PLoS One 2017;12:e0186657.

41. Black PN, Sharpe S. Dietary fat and asthma: is there a connection? Eur Respir J 1997;10:6–12.

42. Woods RK, Thien FC, Abramson MJ. Dietary marine fatty acids (fish oil) for asthma in adults and children. Cochrane Database Syst Rev 2002;(3):CD001283.

43. Gunaratne AW, Makrides M, Collins CT. Maternal prenatal and/or postnatal n-3 long chain polyunsaturated fatty acids (LCPUFA) supplementation for preventing allergies in early childhood. Cochrane Database Syst Rev 2015;(7):CD010085.

44. Hansen S, Strøm M, Maslova E, et al. Fish oil supplementation during pregnancy and allergic respiratory disease in the adult offspring. J Allergy Clin Immunol 2017;139:104–11.e4.

45. Bisgaard H, Stokholm J, Chawes BL, et al. Fish oil-derived fatty acids in pregnancy and wheeze and asthma in offspring. N Engl J Med 2016;375:2530–9.

46. Neutze D, Evans KL, Koenig M, et al. PURLs: does fish oil during pregnancy help prevent asthma in kids? J Fam Pract 2018;67:100–2.
47. Blatter J, Han YY, Forno E, et al. Folate and asthma. Am J Respir Crit Care Med 2013;188:12–7.
48. Parr CL, Magnus MC, Karlstad Ø, et al. Maternal folate intake during pregnancy and childhood asthma in a population-based cohort. Am J Respir Crit Care Med 2017;195:221–8.
49. Wang T, Zhang HP, Zhang X, et al. Is Folate status a risk factor for asthma or other allergic diseases? Allergy Asthma Immunol Res 2015;7:538–46.
50. Roy A, Kocak M, Hartman TJ, et al. Association of prenatal folate status with early childhood wheeze and atopic dermatitis. Pediatr Allergy Immunol 2018;29: 144–50.
51. Brożek JL, Bousquet J, Agache I, et al. Allergic rhinitis and its impact on asthma (ARIA) guidelines-2016 revision. J Allergy Clin Immunol 2017;140:950–8.
52. Lin J, Wang W, Chen P, et al. Prevalence and risk factors of asthma in mainland China: the CARE study. Respir Med 2018;137:48–54.
53. Woodcock A, Lowe LA, Murray CS, et al. Early life environmental control: effect on symptoms, sensitization, and lung function at age 3 years. Am J Respir Crit Care Med 2004;170:433–9.
54. Cardona V, Luengo O, Labrador-Horrillo M. Immunotherapy in allergic rhinitis and lower airway outcomes. Allergy 2017;72:35–42.
55. Schmitt J, Schwarz K, Stadler E, et al. Allergy immunotherapy for allergic rhinitis effectively prevents asthma: results from a large retrospective cohort study. J Allergy Clin Immunol 2015;136:1511–6.
56. Morjaria JB, Caruso M, Emma R, et al. Treatment of allergic rhinitis as a strategy for preventing asthma. Curr Allergy Asthma Rep 2018;18:23.
57. Grembiale RD, Camporota L, Naty S, et al. Effects of specific immunotherapy in allergic rhinitic individuals with bronchial hyperresponsiveness. Am J Respir Crit Care Med 2000;162:2048–52.
58. Jacobsen L, Niggemann B, Dreborg S, et al. Specific immunotherapy has long-term preventive effect of seasonal and perennial asthma: 10-year follow-up on the PAT study. Allergy 2007;62:943–8.
59. Valovirta E, Petersen TH, Piotrowska T, et al. Results from the 5-year SQ grass sublingual immunotherapy tablet asthma prevention (GAP) trial in children with grass pollen allergy. J Allergy Clin Immunol 2018;141:529–38.e13.
60. Kristiansen M, Dhami S, Netuveli G, et al. Allergen immunotherapy for the prevention of allergy: a systematic review and meta-analysis. Pediatr Allergy Immunol 2017;28:18–29.
61. Lowe AJ, Su JC, Allen KJ, et al. A randomized trial of a barrier lipid replacement strategy for the prevention of atopic dermatitis and allergic sensitization: the PEBBLES pilot study. Br J Dermatol 2018;178:e19–21.
62. du Toit G, Sayre PH, Roberts G, et al. Allergen specificity of early peanut consumption and effect on development of allergic disease in the Learning Early About Peanut Allergy study cohort. J Allergy Clin Immunol 2018;141:1343–53.
63. Beigelman A, Bacharier LB. Early-life respiratory infections and asthma development: role in disease pathogenesis and potential targets for disease prevention. Curr Opin Allergy Clin Immunol 2016;16:172–8.
64. Kwong CG, Bacharier LB. Microbes and the role of antibiotic treatment for wheezy lower respiratory tract illnesses in preschool children. Curr Allergy Asthma Rep 2017;17:34.

65. Bacharier LB, Cohen R, Schweiger T, et al. Determinants of asthma after severe respiratory syncytial virus bronchiolitis. J Allergy Clin Immunol 2012;130: 91–100.e3.

66. Jackson DJ, Gangnon RE, Evans MD, et al. Wheezing rhinovirus illnesses in early life predict asthma development in high-risk children. Am J Respir Crit Care Med 2008;178:667–72.

67. Blanken MO, Rovers MM, Molenaar JM, et al. Respiratory syncytial virus and recurrent wheeze in healthy preterm infants. N Engl J Med 2013;368:1791–9.

68. Scheltema NM, Nibbelke EE, Pouw J, et al. Respiratory syncytial virus prevention and asthma in healthy preterm infants: a randomised controlled trial. Lancet Respir Med 2018;6:257–64.

69. Meissner HC, Kimberlin DW. RSV immunoprophylaxis: does the benefit justify the cost? Pediatrics 2013;132:915–8.

70. Piacentini GL, Peroni DG, Bodini A, et al. Azithromycin reduces bronchial hyperresponsiveness and neutrophilic airway inflammation in asthmatic children: a preliminary report. Allergy Asthma Proc 2007;28:194–8.

71. Beigelman A, Mikols CL, Gunsten SP, et al. Azithromycin attenuates airway inflammation in a mouse model of viral bronchiolitis. Respir Res 2010;11:90.

72. Beigelman A, Isaacson-Schmid M, Sajol G, et al. Randomized trial to evaluate azithromycin's effects on serum and upper airway IL-8 levels and recurrent wheezing in infants with respiratory syncytial virus bronchiolitis. J Allergy Clin Immunol 2015;135:1171–8.e1.

73. Zhou Y, Bacharier LB, Isaacson-Schmid M, et al. Azithromycin therapy during respiratory syncytial virus bronchiolitis: upper airway microbiome alterations and subsequent recurrent wheeze. J Allergy Clin Immunol 2016;138:1215–9.e5.

74. Esposito S, Soto-Martinez ME, Feleszko W, et al. Nonspecific immunomodulators for recurrent respiratory tract infections, wheezing and asthma in children: a systematic review of mechanistic and clinical evidence. Curr Opin Allergy Clin Immunol 2018;18(3):198–209.

75. Razi CH, Harmancı K, Abacı A, et al. The immunostimulant OM-85 BV prevents wheezing attacks in preschool children. J Allergy Clin Immunol 2010;126:763–9.

76. Del-Rio-Navarro BE, Espinosa Rosales F, Flenady V, et al. Immunostimulants for preventing respiratory tract infection in children. Cochrane Database Syst Rev 2006;(4):CD004974.

The Effects of the Environment on Asthma Disease Activity

Margee Louisias, MD, MPH[a,b], Amira Ramadan, MD[c,d],
Ahmad Salaheddine Naja, MD[c,e], Wanda Phipatanakul, MD, MS[a,*]

KEYWORDS

- Asthma • Environment • Allergens • Pollutants • Disparities • Asthma morbidity
- Microbiome • Endotoxin

KEY POINTS

- There are influential factors in the biological, physical, and psychosocial environments of children with asthma. They can be protective or a risk factor for developing asthma depending on the timing of exposure, or they can be a trigger for current asthma.
- Allergen exposure is a significant asthma trigger, and remediation is an important component of asthma management. However, there is a lack of high-quality evidence for single-component interventions.
- Coarse particulate matter has been recently found to be associated with prevalent asthma and asthma health care utilization.
- Social factors are associated with asthma outcomes and should be addressed with law and policy reform.
- More innovative, patient-oriented, and health services research approaches should be considered to further evaluate the environment's role in asthma.

Summary Conflict of Interest Statements for Each Author (or a statement indicating no conflicts exist for the specified author[s]): All authors have no conflicts of interest.

Funding and Support: This article was conducted with the support of grants AHRQ and K12HS022986, NIAID K24AI 106822, U01 AI110397, R01HL137192, U01 AI 126614, R01HL137192, U01 AI 126614, U01 AI 110397, and The Allergy and Asthma Awareness Initiative, Inc.

[a] Division of Allergy and Immunology, Boston Children's Hospital, Harvard Medical School, 300 Longwood Avenue, Fegan Building, 6th floor, Boston, MA 02115, USA; [b] Division of Rheumatology, Immunology and Allergy, Brigham and Women's Hospital, Boston, MA, USA; [c] Division of Allergy and Immunology, Boston Children's Hospital, 300 Longwood Avenue, Fegan Building, 6th Floor, Boston, MA 02115, USA; [d] Beth Israel Deaconess Medical Center, Boston, MA; [e] Lebanese American University, Beirut, Lebanon
* Corresponding author.
E-mail address: Wanda.Phipatanakul@childrens.harvard.edu

INTRODUCTION

Asthma is one of the most common chronic conditions in children with, the highest prevalence rates among Puerto Ricans and blacks and minority communities.[1,2] It is associated with significant morbidity, health care utilization, and productivity loss.[1,3,4] Despite advances in asthma therapies and health insurance expansion,[5] the biologic, physical, and psychosocial environment can still impact asthma disease activity.[6]

Understanding influential factors in the biologic, physical, and psychosocial environments of children with asthma is integral to managing asthma. This article highlights current evidence and advances regarding the role of environmental elements affecting asthma activity, through a determinants of health lens.[7]

BIOLOGICAL, PHYSICAL, AND PSYCHOSOCIAL ENVIRONMENTS

The determinants of health framework approach to the role of the environment in asthma, can be thought of in 3 categories: biologic, physical and psychosocial environments.[8,9]

BIOLOGIC ENVIRONMENT

Over the past 2 decades, there has been increased attention to the role of the indoor environment (eg, work, home, or school) in asthma management. Exposure to multiple indoor allergens in US homes is common. In a cross-sectional study, more than half of surveyed homes had detectable levels of all allergens (dust mite, dog, cat, cockroach, mouse, and *Alternaria alternata*), and most homes had at least 3 allergens at increased levels.[10] Multiple studies have shown that indoor allergens, biologic matter, and pollutants including mouse, cockroach, pets, dust mite, mold, endotoxin, and nitrogen dioxide are important asthma symptom risk factors in homes and schools.[11] Simons and colleagues[12] demonstrated in a study of 120 inner-city homes of children with asthma that the high airborne pollutant levels and inner-city home characteristics predisposed them to greater asthma morbidity. In addition to home, children with asthma will have exposures in other environments where they spend time (eg, school).[11,13] The indoor school environment is a reservoir of allergens, molds, pollutants, and endotoxins, and recent studies suggest a significant relationship between school allergen exposure and pediatric asthma morbidity.[14,15] Additionally, there is a paucity of high-quality evidence regarding single-component interventions and indoor allergen exposure reduction and asthma outcomes.[16]

Allergens

Dust mites
Dust mites are one of the most prevalent sources of indoor allergens and the most studied allergen in asthma development.[17] The most common dust mite species are Der f 1 (*Dermatophagoides farinae*) and Der p 2 (*Dermatophagoides pteronyssinus*). Dust mite allergens activate the adaptive and innate immune systems,[18] and Der f 1 induces inflammatory cell death in bronchial epithelial cells.[19] Almost 85% of allergic asthmatic children are sensitized to either or both dust mite species.[20] In children who are sensitized to dust mite, dust mite exposure is associated with increased bronchial hyper-responsiveness, impaired respiratory function, and increased inflammation.[21]

Strategies to reduce dust mite include: frequent washing of all bed linens in hot water, use of allergen-impermeable mattresses and pillow encasements, and measures targeting other dust mite reservoirs such as vacuuming and removal of carpet and stuffed toys. Of note, there is no recent evidence suggesting modern carpets do not serve as a dust mite allergen reservoir.[22] Dust mite acaricides can reduce dust mite allergen burden but are not associated with improvement in pulmonary physiology or asthma symptoms, when compared with placebo or when part of multicomponent interventions.[16] Maintaining indoor humidity at 35% to 50% can reduce dust mite proliferation and survival but can be difficult to sustain. Moreover, high-efficiency particulate air (HEPA) filtration has not been shown to have a great effect on lessening dust mite exposure.[21]

Rodents (mouse)

The major mouse allergen, Mus m 1, is excreted in mouse urine and found in dander and hair follicles. Mus m 1 is carried on small particles, and remains airborne for prolonged periods of time. It is found in house dust particles and is high in kitchens, but also found in bedrooms.[23] Mus m 1 was previously thought to be a significant occupational exposure but is now known to have a role in asthma morbidity.[24] Recent studies demonstrate a high prevalence of mouse allergen in domestic households, where urban homes have higher mouse allergen levels compared with suburban and rural homes. Patient report of rodent infestation has a high positive predictive value for high home mouse allergen levels,[25] but a negative report is not reliable for ruling out exposure.[26]

Although dust mite is the most common allergen sensitization in children with asthma, new literature suggests mouse allergen is the most relevant urban allergen, more than cockroach allergen.[27] Mouse allergen had the highest rate of detection in homes and schools but was significantly higher in schools in the School Inner-City Asthma Study. Mouse allergen exposure, independent of sensitization and home allergen exposure, was significantly associated with more asthma symptoms days and decreased forced expiratory volume in 1 second percentage (FEV_1%) predicted, suggesting the school environment's importance in urban asthma. An ongoing school-specific environmental intervention is being conducted, targeting exposures including mouse (NCT02291302).[15,28]

The Mouse Allergen and Asthma Intervention Trial investigated if professionally delivered integrated pest management and education compared with education alone was associated with improved asthma morbidity. No difference was found, and there was no statistically significant difference in the proportion of subjects with large decreases of mouse allergen (except for 1 airborne measure) between groups. Results were limited, as both arms had significant reductions in exposure, limiting the ability to detect a difference and inability to double blind the environmental intervention.[29]

Cockroach

Cockroach allergy has been established as an important cause of asthma exacerbations for the past few decades. The German cockroach (*Blattella germanica*) and American cockroach (*Periplaneta americana*) are the most medically important species. Cockroach allergens Bla g 1 and Bla g 2 are mostly evaluated in exposure assessment studies.[30]

Recent evidence based on skin prick testing, found that 60% to 80% of inner-city children with asthma are sensitized to cockroach. A study in 61 homes of low-income Chicago children also found that cockroach allergen exposure in bedrooms was associated with increased asthma symptoms.[31] Although less investigated, cockroach allergen is also detectable in suburban and rural homes, albeit at lower concentrations.

Two components to cockroach allergen remediation are suppression of cockroach populations and removal of the residual cockroach allergen.[32] The New Orleans Roach Elimination Study was a randomized trial examining the effect of cockroach insecticidal bait on asthma symptom days. Interestingly, the intervention effect was associated with cockroach sensitization. Cockroach sensitized children in the control group had a significantly higher number of missed school days, symptom days, and health care utilization.[33] Notably cockroach numbers significantly reduced and stayed low for 6 to 12 months, but symptoms gradually improved over 6 to 12 months. This lag in symptom improvement has been attributed to the cockroach allergen in cracks, crevices and walls, suggesting professional cleaning and abatement are critical to comprehensive cockroach management.[34,35]

Cat and dog

Cat and dog are the most common indoor furry pets, and sensitization is known to be associated with severe asthma in childhood.[36] Allergic sensitization to cat and dog is quite common; approximately 12% of the general population and 25% to 65% of children with persistent asthma are sensitized to cat or dog allergens.[37] Fel d 1 and Can f 1 are the major allergens for cat and dog, respectively, and are present in saliva, hair follicles, and skin. Pet allergens are predominantly carried on small particles (<10–20 mm), allowing them to remain airborne for long periods of time and adhere to clothing and surfaces. Therefore, pet allergens are carried long distances, and are passively transferred to environments where no pets are present, leading to indirect exposure[35–39] Children in classes with greater than 18% cat owners had a ninefold increased risk of exacerbated asthma after school started compared with children in classes with no more than 18% cat owners.[40]

The ideal approach furry pet allergen exposure reduction is to remove the pet from the home. The only study examining pet removal demonstrated that by 20 to 24 weeks after cat removal, most homes with pet cats had cat allergen levels similar to control homes without cats.[41] Control of cat allergen exposure is accomplished by: pet removal from the home/bedroom; regular cleaning allergen reservoirs (upholstered furniture, walls, and carpet), encase the mattress and pillows with bed encasing (pore diameter <6 μm), regular pet washing and HEPA filtration.[35,42]

Mold

There is a wide variety of indoor and outdoor molds, and their allergenic proteins vary by mold species. The most common species to which children are sensitized and exposed are *Alternaria* and *Cladosporium* (outdoor), *Aspergillus*, and *Penicillium* (indoor).[43] The prevalence of mold sensitization in children with persistent asthma is variable in the literature, ranging from 12% to 66%.[44,45] Qualitative assessments of fungal exposure in the form of mildew odor or visible mold have been linked to increased risk of allergic rhinitis and asthma.[46] Furthermore, a recent study by Baxi and colleagues[47] demonstrated that the school/classroom environment can be a source of mold exposure, both in quantity of spores and variety of mold types, and the presence of visible mold may be a predictor of high mold spore counts.

Mold exposure can contribute to severe asthma and to asthma development. Mold-sensitized children have significantly lower lung function and increased airway hyper-responsiveness compared with children not sensitized to mold.[43,44,48,49] Birth cohorts have demonstrated a relationship between mold sensitization and recurrent wheezing and asthma and a recent birth cohort study in Boston revealed a significant relationship between indoor dust-borne *Alternaria* at the age of 2 to 3 months and the frequency of wheeze by 1 year old, even after adjustment for outdoor airborne *Alternaria* concentrations.[50–52]

There are no solitary or randomized controlled trials of mold remediation. Mold remediation has only been included in multicomponent strategies (eg, interventions also targeting dust mites or furry pet allergens), which have all shown improved asthma symptoms.[16] Mold remediation includes: mold removal from surfaces (using cleaner and fungicide), repair of leaky water sources, dehumidification, and ventilator system installation. Mold remediation can be costly and burdensome. Chew and colleagues[53] proposed a 2-part interview to guide clinicians on how to decide which patients would warrant in-home assessments for mold exposure with an indoor environment professional (IEP). Presently, the literature insufficiently explains which children would be at risk for developing asthma from mold exposure or if there is a dose threshold of mold exposure that will exacerbate asthma.

Endotoxin

Endotoxin is part of the gram-negative bacteria's outer membrane and is shed after bacteria die.[54] Endotoxin induces airway inflammation via Toll-like receptor (TLR) 4 and is an established asthma risk factor. Higher domestic endotoxin levels are linked to increased asthma prevalence, severity, and exacerbations.

Endotoxin in homes has been demonstrated to increase wheeze[55] and can potentiate the airway response to allergens in people with asthma.[56] A cross-sectional study found: poverty, Mexican ethnicity, younger age, carpeting, furry pet, cockroaches, and/or a household smoker predicted higher endotoxin levels.[57] Endotoxin in other indoor areas such as the school also has an impact on asthma morbidity. Sheehan and colleagues[58] identified higher settled-dust endotoxin levels in inner-city schools compared with students' homes. In this same cohort, classroom-specific airborne endotoxin levels were found to be independently associated with increased asthma symptoms in children with nonatopic asthma, after adjusting for home exposures.[59]

Conversely, there is also literature supporting the contrary, that early endotoxin exposure is protective of childhood asthma.[60–62] Endotoxin's protective qualities were recently highlighted by Stein and colleagues[60] in their investigations of environmental exposures, ancestry, and immune profiles of Amish and Hutterite children. None of the Amish children and 20% of the Hutterite children had asthma. The Amish homes had significantly higher median levels of endotoxin in airborne dust compared with the Hutterite homes, respectively. Endotoxin's protective and exacerbative roles in asthma underscore that the timing of exposures plays a critical role in asthma.

Microbiome

The microbiome is the combination of all microbes colonizing skin and mucosal surfaces, their genomic elements, and interactions.[63] Many factors play a role in influencing the development, evolution, and stability of the microbiome, such as the innate immune response, genetic factors and environmental factors (eg, dietary factors, antibiotics, and infections).[64] Any disruption in this stability can increase risk of allergic diseases later in life.

Several studies have linked early life dysbiosis or microbial imbalance in the gut microbiota with an altered risk of asthma later in life.[65] Arrieta and colleagues,[66] reported that the first 100 days may be a critical window for the impact of microbial dysbiosis and the risk of atopic wheezing in early childhood. This linkage has been attributed to the gut-lung axis due to cross-talk between gut and lung microbiota.[67] More specifically, the gut microbiota can influence the lung immune response by production of bacterial ligands, bacterial metabolites (eg, short-chain fatty acids, histamine), and immune cells.

Similar to the gut microbiome, the lung microbiota can affect innate and adaptive immune responses in the lung, by its interaction with airway epithelium and immune cells. The upper and lower airway microbiome is a complex niche of diverse microbes that play a role in asthma.[63] Some specific phylum have been shown to be more prevalent in asthmatic patients. For example, patients with uncontrolled asthma showed a greater microbiota diversity compared with control subjects; this diversity correlated positively with bronchial hyperresponsiveness.[68] Teo and colleagues demonstrated that nasopharyngeal aspirates, collected by 7 weeks of age and younger, with greater than 20% *Streptococcus* colonization, were associated with a 4 times increased odds of chronic wheeze at 5 years old. A 2018 observational study concluded several important points relating microbiome and asthma.[69] First, gut microbiome maturation during the first year of life is important. Second, there is a potential beneficial effect of specific microbial supplementation in the first year of life in children at high risk of developing asthma. Third, gut microbiome immaturity in the first year of life is a critical determinant for increased asthma risk.

Despite the current evidence, it is unclear whether the changes in the microbiome are a result of having asthma or are causative of asthma.

Recent data from Lai and colleagues[70] suggest that external microbiomes matter also. This study found that the composition of the home and school microbiomes significantly differed, and the classroom microbial diversity was associated with a significantly increased odds of asthma symptom days. Additionally, integrated pest management and not HEPA filtration changed classroom microbial community structure.

Genetics

Genetic variants and epigenetic changes are likely contributors to the origins of asthma, source of phenotypic variability, and response to therapy.[71–73] There is evidence that complex gene–environment interactions as seen in the increased risk of asthma in offspring of mothers who smoked during pregnancy and 17q21 variants are strongly associated with childhood asthma.[74] Despite the progress in genetic research, understanding is still limited, as these genetic factors explain a small proportion of total phenotypic variability, and the functional relationships between epigenetic processes, environmental stimuli, and developmental programs.[75] Farzan and colleagues[76] examined the association of the rs7216389 (17q21 single SNP) with health care utilization and oral steroid bursts from the Pharmacogenetics in Childhood Asthma consortium. The rs7216389 SNP was significantly associated with asthma emergency room visits and admissions and use of oral steroid bursts. Nevertheless, current studies of human allergy and asthma epigenetics have primarily focused on concurrent disease,[71] showing DNA methylation marks in specific gene loci are associated with asthma and epigenetic changes might play a role in establishing the asthma phenotype.[77]

DNA methylation changes in genes with direct relevance to Th2 immunity and asthma are associated with allergic asthma in African American inner-city children.[77] The IL4Rα-Q576R polymorphism is associated with asthma prevalence and severity. The IL4Rα-Q576R genotype was recently found to be an effect modifier of the association between urban classroom endotoxin levels and asthma symptoms days,[78] demonstrating gene-environment interaction.

Innate immunity genes (CD14, TLR4, and TLR2, the critical mediators of responses to bacteria in the extracellular space) also play a prominent role among gene-environment interaction studies of asthma-related phenotypes.[79]

PHYSICAL ENVIRONMENT
Air Pollution

Air pollution is an ubiquitous combination of pollutants including particulate matter (PM), chemical and biological materials like carbon monoxide (CO), nitrogen dioxide (NO_2), black carbon (CO), and sulfur dioxide (SO_2).[80] There is a multitude of evidence that ambient air pollution can exacerbate pre-existing asthma. Exposure to high levels of NO_2, $PM_{2.5}$ (aerodynamic diameter of 2.5 microns or less) and CO are associated with increased differentially methylated regions of the Foxp3 gene promoter region, which was shown to be significantly associated with asthma.[81] A 2017 meta-analysis investigated the association between outdoor air pollution and asthma exacerbations, taking into consideration lag times between air pollution increase and asthma exacerbations.[82] In the subgroup analysis of children, asthma exacerbations were significantly associated with higher concentration of NO_2, SO_2, and $PM_{2.5}$. Even short-term exposure to ozone, NO_2, or SO_2 can increase children's asthma symptoms.[83] Another study revealed a significant association between traffic-related air pollution exposure and higher hospital readmission rates.[84] Such findings are critical for inner-city schools because of their close proximity to highways, heavy traffic, and industrial buildings. These establishments tend to be located centrally, among condensed traffic, with sites of idling cars increasing air pollution within and around the school.[83–85]

NO_2 is generated from fossil fuel combustion in homes and outdoors but can be found in other settings. Gaffin and colleagues[86] showed a nonsignificant temporally distinct association of NO_2 levels measured in inner-city school classrooms with airflow obstruction in children with asthma. This concordance was attributed to NO_2 having adverse effects on health outcomes at levels undetected by the existing standards in a susceptible population.

PM is comprised of airborne particles expressed as either $PM_{2.5}$ or $PM_{10-2.5}$ (aerodynamic diameter more than 2.5 microns to 10 microns). $PM_{2.5}$ is associated with worsening asthma symptoms and increased oxidative stress based on inflammation biomarkers.[84] Bouazza and colleagues[87] found an association between $PM_{2.5}$ and pediatric emergency department visits. There are fewer data on the long-term consequences of $PM_{10-2.5}$ because of the lack of monitoring locations for both PM_{10} and $PM_{2.5}$. Additionally, $PM_{10-2.5}$ is thought to be less harmful than $PM_{2.5}$, as its size may limit its lung penetration, but Keet and colleagues[88] found that $PM_{10-2.5}$ was associated with increased asthma prevalence and health care utilization.

PSYCHOSOCIAL ENVIRONMENT

The psychosocial environment is becoming increasingly recognized[89] as a significant contributor to asthma morbidity.[9,90] It includes a person's neighborhood, socioeconomic status, family relationships, and social networks. Kopel and colleagues[91] demonstrated that the primary caregiver's perception of neighborhood safety is associated with childhood asthma morbidity among inner-city schoolchildren with asthma, and caregiver stress is related to asthma morbidity among children.[89] Census tract-level violent and all-crime rates have also been associated with population-level rates of asthma utilization (emergency department and admissions[92]).

Chen and colleagues[93] investigated whether living in areas high in greenspace would help balance the effects of difficult family relationship for children with asthma. A synergistic effect of positive family relationships across the physical and social domains was seen, and children with asthma benefited the most when they lived in high greenspace areas and had positive family relationships. Discrimination has also been recently evaluated as a contributor to poor outcomes in medical conditions. Thakur and colleagues[89] investigated the association between perceived discrimination and asthma status and morbidity in black and Latino youth with asthma. Blacks reporting any severity of discrimination had a 78% increased odds of having asthma and 97% increased odds of poor asthma control.

Structural discrimination can impact asthma as it can manifest as unequal access to high-quality medical resources, substandard housing,[94] lack of homeownership, and living in neighborhoods with higher levels of pollution (eg, closer proximity to highways, pollutant-producing factories[95]).

The 2011 American Housing Survey was analyzed by Hughes and colleagues, who found that poor housing quality was significantly associated with asthma diagnosis and emergency department visits. Home ownership was associated with lower odds of asthma emergency department visits.

These findings highlight that efforts to improve asthma outcomes should include social support and services and law and policy change.

SUMMARY

Asthma continues to be a significant cause of morbidity in children. The child's environment is integral to asthma development and activity. This review article focused on the most recent evidence supporting the role of environment in asthma disease activity from biologic, physical, and psychosocial perspectives. The evidence supports that some environmental exposures can be protective or a risk factor for asthma depending on exposure timing. Regarding future directions, it is important to investigate the critical exposure windows in pregnancy, childhood, and adulthood through cohort studies and randomized trials. Consideration of pragmatic study designs may allow increased recruitment. There is also a need to improve evidence for single-component allergen remediation interventions and to understand which multifaceted intervention combinations have the best synergistic effects. Law and policy reform are also crucial to reduce pollutant exposures, and to address social factors contributing to poor outcomes. Health services research should be utilized to form the evidence base policymakers seek for their decisions. Lastly, more innovative and patient-oriented interventions are needed to evaluate the environment's role.

REFERENCES

1. Most recent asthma data. Available at: https://www.cdc.gov/asthma/most_recent_data.htm. Accessed July 5, 2018.
2. Szentpetery SE, Forno E, Canino G, et al. Asthma in Puerto Ricans: lessons from a high-risk population. J Allergy Clin Immunol 2016;138:1556–8.
3. Akinbami LJ, Simon AE, Rossen LM. Changing trends in asthma prevalence among children. Pediatrics 2016;137.
4. Asthma-related missed school days among children aged 5–17 years. 2015;3(1). Available at: https://www.cdc.gov/asthma/asthma_stats/missing_days.htm. Accessed July 5, 2018.
5. Sommers BD, Gawande AA, Baicker K. Health insurance coverage and health—what the recent evidence tells us. N Engl J Med 2017;377(6):586–93.
6. Gleason M, Cicutto L, Haas-Howard C, et al. Leveraging partnerships: families, schools, and providers working together to improve asthma management. Curr Allergy Asthma Rep 2016;16:74.

7. Determinants of Health. *Healthcare-Associated Infections | Healthy People 2020*, US Department of Health and Human Services, 2014. Available at: www.healthypeople. gov/2020/about/foundation-health-measures/Determinants-of-Health.

8. Bearer CF. Environmental health hazards: how children are different from adults. Future Child 1995;5:11–26.

9. Chen E, Schreier HM. Does the social environment contribute to asthma? Immunol Allergy Clin North Am 2008;28:649–64.

10. Salo PM, Arbes SJ, Crockett PW, et al. Exposure to multiple indoor allergens in US homes and its relationship to asthma. J Allergy Clin Immunol 2008;121: 678–84. e2.

11. Kanchongkittiphon W, Gaffin JM, Phipatanakul W. The indoor environment and inner-city childhood asthma. Asian Pac J Allergy Immunol 2014;32:103–10.

12. Simons E, Curtin-Brosnan J, Buckley T, et al. Indoor environmental differences between inner city and suburban homes of children with asthma. J Urban Health 2007;84:577–90.

13. Permaul P, Hoffman E, Fu C, et al. Allergens in urban schools and homes of children with asthma. Pediatr Allergy Immunol 2012;23:543–9.

14. Esty B, Phipatanakul W. School exposure and asthma. Ann Allergy Asthma Immunol 2018;120(5):482–7.

15. Sheehan WJ, Permaul P, Petty CR, et al. Association between allergen exposure in inner-city schools and asthma morbidity among students. JAMA Pediatr 2017; 171:31–8.

16. Leas BF, D'Anci KE, Apter AJ, et al. Effectiveness of indoor allergen reduction in asthma management: a systematic review. J Allergy Clin Immunol 2018;141: 1854–69.

17. Gaffin JM, Phipatanakul W. The role of indoor allergens in the development of asthma. Curr Opin Allergy Clin Immunol 2009;9:128–35.

18. Calderon MA, Linneberg A, Kleine-Tebbe J, et al. Respiratory allergy caused by house dust mites: what do we really know? J Allergy Clin Immunol 2015;136: 38–48.

19. Tsai YM, Chiang KH, Hung JY, et al. Der f1 induces pyroptosis in human bronchial epithelia via the NLRP3 inflammasome. Int J Mol Med 2018;41:757–64.

20. Wang JY. The innate immune response in house dust mite-induced allergic inflammation. Allergy Asthma Immunol Res 2013;5:68–74.

21. Portnoy J, Miller JD, Williams PB, et al. Environmental assessment and exposure control of dust mites: a practice parameter. Ann Allergy Asthma Immunol 2013; 111:465.

22. Becher R, Ovrevik J, Schwarze PE, et al. Do carpets impair indoor air quality and cause adverse health outcomes: a review. Int J Environ Res Public Health 2018; 15 [pii:E184].

23. Kopel LS, Phipatanakul W, Gaffin JM. Social disadvantage and asthma control in children. Paediatr Respir Rev 2014;15:256–62 [quiz: 262–3].

24. Pongracic JA, Visness CM, Gruchalla RS, et al. Effect of mouse allergen and rodent environmental intervention on asthma in inner-city children. Ann Allergy Asthma Immunol 2008;101:35–41.

25. Loo CK, Foty RG, Wheeler AJ, et al. Do questions reflecting indoor air pollutant exposure from a questionnaire predict direct measure of exposure in owner-occupied houses? Int J Environ Res Public Health 2010;7:3270–97.

26. Phipatanakul W, Matsui E, Portnoy J, et al. Environmental assessment and exposure reduction of rodents: a practice parameter. Ann Allergy Asthma Immunol 2012;109:375–87.

27. Sheehan WJ, Phipatanakul W. Indoor allergen exposure and asthma outcomes. Curr Opin Pediatr 2016;28:772–7.
28. Phipatanakul W, Koutrakis P, Coull BA, et al. The School Inner-City Asthma Intervention Study: design, rationale, methods, and lessons learned. Contemp Clin Trials 2017;60:14–23.
29. Matsui EC, Perzanowski M, Peng RD, et al. Effect of an integrated pest management intervention on asthma symptoms among mouse-sensitized children and adolescents with asthma: a randomized clinical trial. JAMA 2017;317:1027–36.
30. Phipatanakul W. Environmental factors and childhood asthma. Pediatr Ann 2006; 35:646–56.
31. Turyk M, Curtis L, Scheff P, et al. Environmental allergens and asthma morbidity in low-income children. J Asthma 2006;43:453–7.
32. Coleman AT, Rettiganti M, Bai S, et al. Mouse and cockroach exposure in rural Arkansas delta region homes. Ann Allergy Asthma Immunol 2014;112:256–60.
33. Rabito FA, Carlson JC, He H, et al. A single intervention for cockroach control reduces cockroach exposure and asthma morbidity in children. J Allergy Clin Immunol 2017;140:565–70.
34. Portnoy J, Chew GL, Phipatanakul W, et al. Environmental assessment and exposure reduction of cockroaches: a practice parameter. J Allergy Clin Immunol 2013;132:802–8.e1-25.
35. Ahluwalia SK, Matsui EC. Indoor environmental interventions for furry pet allergens, pest allergens, and mold: looking to the future. J Allergy Clin Immunol Pract 2018;6:9–19.
36. Konradsen JR, Nordlund B, Onell A, et al. Severe childhood asthma and allergy to furry animals: refined assessment using molecular-based allergy diagnostics. Pediatr Allergy Immunol 2014;25:187–92.
37. Gergen PJ, Mitchell HE, Calatroni A, et al. Sensitization and exposure to pets: the effect on asthma morbidity in the US population. J Allergy Clin Immunol Pract 2018;6:101–107 e2.
38. Gruchalla RS, Pongracic J, Plaut M, et al. Inner City Asthma Study: relationships among sensitivity, allergen exposure, and asthma morbidity. J Allergy Clin Immunol 2005;115:478–85.
39. Weiss ST, Horner A, Shapiro G, et al. Childhood Asthma Management Program (CAMP) Research Group. The prevalence of environmental exposure to perceived asthma triggers in children with mild-to-moderate asthma: data from the Childhood Asthma Management Program (CAMP). J Allergy Clin Immunol 2001;107:634–40.
40. Almqvist C, Wickman M, Perfetti L, et al. Worsening of asthma in children allergic to cats, after indirect exposure to cat at school. Am J Respir Crit Care Med 2001; 163:694–8.
41. Wood RA, Chapman MD, Adkinson NF Jr, et al. The effect of cat removal on allergen content in household-dust samples. J Allergy Clin Immunol 1989;83: 730–4.
42. Wilson JM, Platts-Mills TAE. Home environmental interventions for house dust mite. J Allergy Clin Immunol Pract 2018;6:1–7.
43. Pongracic JA, O'Connor GT, Muilenberg ML, et al. Differential effects of outdoor versus indoor fungal spores on asthma morbidity in inner-city children. J Allergy Clin Immunol 2010;125:593–9.
44. Byeon JH, Ri S, Amarsaikhan O, et al. Association between sensitization to mold and impaired pulmonary function in children with asthma. Allergy Asthma Immunol Res 2017;9:509–16.

45. O'Driscoll BR, Powell G, Chew F, et al. Comparison of skin prick tests with specific serum immunoglobulin E in the diagnosis of fungal sensitization in patients with severe asthma. Clin Exp Allergy 2009;39:1677–83.

46. Fukutomi Y, Taniguchi M. Sensitization to fungal allergens: resolved and unresolved issues. Allergol Int 2015;64:321–31.

47. Baxi SN, Muilenberg ML, Rogers CA, et al. Exposures to molds in school classrooms of children with asthma. Pediatr Allergy Immunol 2013;24:697–703.

48. Vicencio AG, Santiago MT, Tsirilakis K, et al. Fungal sensitization in childhood persistent asthma is associated with disease severity. Pediatr Pulmonol 2014; 49:8–14.

49. Sharpe RA, Bearman N, Thornton CR, et al. Indoor fungal diversity and asthma: a meta-analysis and systematic review of risk factors. J Allergy Clin Immunol 2015; 135:110–22.

50. Mendell MJ, Mirer AG, Cheung K, et al. Respiratory and allergic health effects of dampness, mold, and dampness-related agents: a review of the epidemiologic evidence. Environ Health Perspect 2011;119:748–56.

51. Behbod B, Sordillo JE, Hoffman EB, et al. Wheeze in infancy: protection associated with yeasts in house dust contrasts with increased risk associated with yeasts in indoor air and other fungal taxa. Allergy 2013;68:1410–8.

52. Halonen M, Stern DA, Wright AL, et al. Alternaria as a major allergen for asthma in children raised in a desert environment. Am J Respir Crit Care Med 1997;155: 1356–61.

53. Chew GL, Horner WE, Kennedy K, et al. Procedures to assist health care providers to determine when home assessments for potential mold exposure are warranted. J Allergy Clin Immunol Pract 2016;4:417–422 e2.

54. Zhu Z, Oh SY, Zheng T, et al. Immunomodulating effects of endotoxin in mouse models of allergic asthma. Clin Exp Allergy 2010;40:536–46.

55. Michel O, Kips J, Duchateau J, et al. Severity of asthma is related to endotoxin in house dust. Am J Respir Crit Care Med 1996;154:1641–6.

56. Boehlecke B, Hazucha M, Alexis NE, et al. Low-dose airborne endotoxin exposure enhances bronchial responsiveness to inhaled allergen in atopic asthmatics. J Allergy Clin Immunol 2003;112:1241–3.

57. Thorne PS, Mendy A, Metwali N, et al. Endotoxin exposure: predictors and prevalence of associated asthma outcomes in the United States. Am J Respir Crit Care Med 2015;192:1287–97.

58. Sheehan WJ, Hoffman EB, Fu C, et al. Endotoxin exposure in inner-city schools and homes of children with asthma. Ann Allergy Asthma Immunol 2012;108: 418–22.

59. Lai PS, Sheehan WJ, Gaffin JM, et al. School endotoxin exposure and asthma morbidity in inner-city children. Chest 2015;148:1251–8.

60. Stein MM, Hrusch CL, Gozdz J, et al. Innate immunity and asthma risk in Amish and Hutterite farm children. N Engl J Med 2016;375:411–21.

61. Karvonen AM, Hyvarinen A, Gehring U, et al. Exposure to microbial agents in house dust and wheezing, atopic dermatitis and atopic sensitization in early childhood: a birth cohort study in rural areas. Clin Exp Allergy 2012;42:1246–56.

62. O'Connor GT, Lynch SV, Bloomberg GR, et al. Early-life home environment and risk of asthma among inner-city children. J Allergy Clin Immunol 2018;141: 1468–75.

63. Sokolowska M, Frei R, Lunjani N, et al. Microbiome and asthma. Asthma Res Pract 2018;4:1.

64. Chung KF. Airway microbial dysbiosis in asthmatic patients: a target for prevention and treatment? J Allergy Clin Immunol 2017;139:1071–81.

65. Kloepfer KM, Sarsani VK, Poroyko V, et al. Community-acquired rhinovirus infection is associated with changes in the airway microbiome. J Allergy Clin Immunol 2017;140:312–315 e8.

66. Arrieta MC, Stiemsma LT, Dimitriu PA, et al. Early infancy microbial and metabolic alterations affect risk of childhood asthma. Sci Transl Med 2015;7:307ra152.

67. Arrieta MC, Arevalo A, Stiemsma L, et al. Associations between infant fungal and bacterial dysbiosis and childhood atopic wheeze in a nonindustrialized setting. J Allergy Clin Immunol 2018;142(2):424–34.e10.

68. Di Cicco M, Pistello M, Jacinto T, et al. Does lung microbiome play a causal or casual role in asthma? Pediatr Pulmonol 2018;53(10):1340–5.

69. Stokholm J, Blaser MJ, Thorsen J, et al. Maturation of the gut microbiome and risk of asthma in childhood. Nat Commun 2018;9:141.

70. Lai PS, Kolde R, Franzosa EA, et al. The classroom microbiome and asthma morbidity in children attending 3 inner-city schools. J Allergy Clin Immunol 2018;141:2311–3.

71. Devries A, Vercelli D. Epigenetics of human asthma and allergy: promises to keep. Asian Pac J Allergy Immunol 2013;31:183–9.

72. Arathimos R, Suderman M, Sharp GC, et al. Epigenome-wide association study of asthma and wheeze in childhood and adolescence. Clin Epigenetics 2017;9:112.

73. Barton SJ, Ngo S, Costello P, et al. DNA methylation of Th2 lineage determination genes at birth is associated with allergic outcomes in childhood. Clin Exp Allergy 2017;47:1599–608.

74. Ramadas RA, Sadeghnejad A, Karmaus W, et al. Interleukin-1R antagonist gene and pre-natal smoke exposure are associated with childhood asthma. Eur Respir J 2007;29:502–8.

75. DeVries A, Vercelli D. Early predictors of asthma and allergy in children: the role of epigenetics. Curr Opin Allergy Clin Immunol 2015;15:435–9.

76. Farzan N, Vijverberg SJ, Hernandez-Pacheco N, et al. 17q21 variant increases the risk of exacerbations in asthmatic children despite inhaled corticosteroids use. Allergy 2018;73(10):2083–8.

77. Yang IV, Pedersen BS, Liu A, et al. DNA methylation and childhood asthma in the inner city. J Allergy Clin Immunol 2015;136:69–80.

78. Lai PS, Massoud AH, Xia M, et al. Gene-environment interaction between an IL4R variant and school endotoxin exposure contributes to asthma symptoms in inner-city children. J Allergy Clin Immunol 2018;141:794–6.e3.

79. Vercelli D. Gene-environment interactions in asthma and allergy: the end of the beginning? Curr Opin Allergy Clin Immunol 2010;10:145–8.

80. Mannucci PM, Harari S, Martinelli I, et al. Effects on health of air pollution: a narrative review. Intern Emerg Med 2015;10:657–62.

81. Prunicki M, Stell L, Dinakarpandian D, et al. Exposure to NO_2, CO, and $PM_{2.5}$ is linked to regional DNA methylation differences in asthma. Clin Epigenetics 2018;10:2.

82. Orellano P, Quaranta N, Reynoso J, et al. Effect of outdoor air pollution on asthma exacerbations in children and adults: systematic review and multilevel meta-analysis. PloS One 2017;12:e0174050.

83. Naja A, Phipatanakul W, Permaul P. Taming asthma in school-aged children: a comprehensive review. J Allergy Clin Immunol 2018;6(3):726–35.

84. Pollock J, Shi L, Gimbel RW. Outdoor environment and pediatric asthma: an update on the evidence from North America. Can Respir J 2017;2017:8921917.
85. Yoda Y, Takagi H, Wakamatsu J, et al. Acute effects of air pollutants on pulmonary function among students: a panel study in an isolated island. Environ Health Prev Med 2017;22:33.
86. Gaffin JM, Hauptman M, Petty CR, et al. Nitrogen dioxide exposure in school classrooms of inner-city children with asthma. J Allergy Clin Immunol 2018; 141(6):2249–55.e2.
87. Bouazza N, Foissac F, Urien S, et al. Fine particulate pollution and asthma exacerbations. Arch Dis Child 2018;103(9):828–31.
88. Keet CA, Keller JP, Peng RD. Long-term coarse particulate matter exposure is associated with asthma among children in Medicaid. Am J Respir Crit Care Med 2018;197:737–46.
89. Thakur N, Barcelo NE, Borrell LN, et al. Perceived discrimination associated with asthma and related outcomes in minority youth: the GALA II and SAGE II studies. Chest 2017;151:804–12.
90. Williams DR, Sternthal M, Wright RJ. Social determinants: taking the social context of asthma seriously. Pediatrics 2009;123:S174–84.
91. Kopel LS, Gaffin JM, Ozonoff A, et al. Perceived neighborhood safety and asthma morbidity in the School Inner-City Asthma Study. Pediatr Pulmonol 2015;50: 17–24.
92. Beck AF, Huang B, Ryan PH, et al. Areas with high rates of police-reported violent crime have higher rates of childhood asthma morbidity. J Pediatr 2016;173: 175–82. e1.
93. Chen E, Miller GE, Shalowitz MU, et al. Difficult family relationships, residential greenspace, and childhood asthma. Pediatrics 2017;139 [pii:e20163056].
94. Mehta AJ, Dooley DP, Kane J, et al. Subsidized housing and adult asthma in Boston, 2010–2015. Am J Public Health 2018;108(8):1059–65.
95. Shamasunder B, Collier-Oxandale A, Blickley J, et al. Community-based health and exposure study around urban oil developments in south Los Angeles. Int J Environ Res Public Health 2018;15:138.

Management of Asthma in the Preschool Child

Christina G. Kwong, MD, Leonard B. Bacharier, MD*

KEYWORDS

- Asthma • Therapy • Preschool child • Antibacterial agents

KEY POINTS

- Asthma in the preschool age group consists of heterogeneous phenotypes, which may exhibit differential responses to treatment approaches.
- A severe intermittent wheeze phenotype is commonly seen in the preschool population.
- A variety of treatment strategies have been demonstrated to decrease severe episodes in the severe intermittent wheeze phenotype.
- Preschool children with persistent asthma with evidence of aeroallergen sensitization and/ or peripheral blood eosinophilia should be started on daily low-dose inhaled corticosteroids as initial therapy.

INTRODUCTION

Just 1 or 2 decades ago, asthma management in the preschool age group of 1- to 5-year-old children primarily consisted of approaches extrapolated from older children. We have come a long way since then, although this age group continues to be a challenging population to manage. Morbidity is also high; health care use for asthma during childhood is greatest among the 0- to 4-year-old group.[1]

Although it is common for preschool children to wheeze during the first year of life, only a subset will go on to have recurrent or persistent wheezing (ie, asthma).[2,3] A diagnosis of asthma in this age group requires consideration of multiple early life host and environmental factors, and symptoms can have multiple trajectories of disease expression and response to therapy.[2,4] Several early life wheezing and asthma phenotypes have been identified, and these phenotypes have distinct, but often overlapping, characteristics. Children may switch between phenotypes or evolve into

Disclosure Statement: C.G. Kwong: No financial or commercial interests to disclose. L.B. Bacharier: Dr Bacharier reports grants from NIH; personal fees from GlaxoSmithKline, Genentech/Novartis, Merck, DBV Technologies, Teva, Boehringer Ingelheim, AstraZeneca, WebMD/Medscape, Sanofi/Regeneron, Vectura, and Circassia.
Department of Pediatrics, Washington University School of Medicine in St. Louis, Campus Box 8116, 660 South Euclid Avenue, St Louis, MO 63110, USA
* Corresponding author.
E-mail address: Bacharier_l@wustl.edu

another. Furthermore, the phenotypes may affect management decisions or response to specific therapies.

In this review, the authors discuss current management strategies for asthma in the preschool population.

MANAGEMENT BASED ON CURRENT KNOWLEDGE OF EARLY LIFE PHENOTYPES
Based on Status of Atopy and Allergic Sensitization

Children with evidence of atopy or allergic sensitization

Several phenotypic characterizations relating to atopy and allergic sensitization have been found to be associated with differences in response to asthma therapies in this age group. The first, and most widely used, is the Asthma Predictive Index, particularly the modified version (mAPI).[5,6] This index is used for children during the first 3 years of life to help predict the likelihood of persistent asthma at age 6 years, increasing the posttest probability to 90% in a high-risk cohort.[7] The mAPI is positive if a child has had at least 4 episodes of wheezing in 1 year in addition to having at least 1 major or 2 minor criteria. The major criteria are:

1. Parental asthma, physician diagnosed,
2. Atopic dermatitis, physician diagnosed, or
3. Allergic sensitization to an aeroallergen.

The minor criteria are:

1. Wheezing unrelated to colds,
2. Blood eosinophil levels of at least 4%, and
3. Allergic sensitization to milk, egg, or peanut.

The mAPI differs from the original form in that allergic sensitization to 1 or more aeroallergens is added as a major criterion, and the minor criterion of physician-diagnosed allergic rhinitis is replaced by allergic sensitization to milk, egg, or peanuts.

If a child has a positive mAPI, the preferred initial treatment option is a daily inhaled corticosteroid (ICS), which has been shown to be an effective therapy in the preschool age group in general and particularly among preschoolers with a positive mAPI.[8-11] The Prevention of Early Asthma in Kids (PEAK) trial enrolled 285 children 2 to 3 years of age[6] with a positive mAPI. Those with persistent symptoms during a run-in period were excluded. Participants were randomized to active treatment with either inhaled low-dose fluticasone propionate 88 mcg twice daily or placebo for 2 years, and then the treatment was stopped with continued outcome monitoring for 12 months. In this trial, daily ICS use was associated with a greater number of symptom-free days and fewer exacerbations during the 2 years of active therapy.[9] Furthermore, in a post hoc subgroup analysis, ICS use in those with a positive mAPI was associated with more symptom-free days and fewer exacerbations if the participants were male, Caucasian, had an asthma-related emergency department (ED) visit or hospitalization within the past year, or had sensitization to an aeroallergen.[12] These findings highlight that even within the positive mAPI group, there remains substantial heterogeneity in ICS treatment response.

Components of the mAPI have also been found to be associated with a greater response to daily ICS therapy. In the Individualized Therapy for Asthma in Toddlers study (INFANT), which featured a crossover design, children aged 12 to 59 months of age who were candidates for step 2 therapy (ie, daily controller) were enrolled to assess the differential response to daily ICS, intermittent ICS whenever a short-acting beta-agonist was used, and a daily leukotriene receptor antagonist (LTRA).[13] All participants were treated with 16 weeks of each therapy in a randomized order. Asthma control was most likely to be best during the daily ICS treatment periods, and this finding was further increased in the patients with aeroallergen sensitization or blood eosinophil counts of at least 300/μL. Overall, based on the results of this study and because ICS has been shown to be the most effective therapy overall, preschoolers requiring daily controller therapy (step 2) with evidence of aeroallergen sensitization and/or blood eosinophil levels of at least 300/μL should be started on daily low-dose ICS as first-line therapy (**Fig. 1**).

Children without evidence of atopy or allergic sensitization
In the INFANT study described elsewhere in this article, 26% of the participants did not demonstrate a preference for any of the 3 therapies and were called nondifferential responders. After incorporating this subgroup into the analysis, the probability of a best response to ICS was less than 40% for the entire cohort,[13] suggesting that there is a significant subgroup of patients for whom daily ICS is not the most likely to be effective, and comparable proportions of these patients responded best to either montelukast or intermittent ICS. In this study, the investigators were unable to identify predictors of best response to LTRA or intermittent ICS. Children who were not sensitized to aeroallergens and had blood eosinophil levels less than 300/μL experienced similar (and relatively low) exacerbation rates during treatment with all 3 approaches. Based on these findings, children without features suggestive of atopy with persistent symptoms and/or recurrent exacerbations who are candidates for step 2 therapy can be started on either a daily ICS, LTRA, or intermittent, symptom-driven ICS.

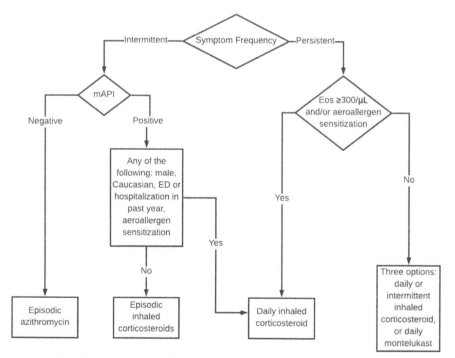

Fig. 1. Preferred treatments based on phenotypes. ED, emergency department; Eos, eosinophils; mAPI, modified asthma predictive index.

The decision as to which therapy should include consideration of these findings and provider and/or parent preferences.

Based on Symptom Pattern or Trigger

A characteristic of many preschool wheezers is that they experience acute episodes of severe disease, typically associated with viral illnesses, interspersed between prolonged asymptomatic periods.[14–16] This subgroup has been referred to by several terms, including recurrent viral wheeze, episodic viral wheeze, and severe intermittent wheeze. The latter was characterized in the Acute Intervention Management Strategies (AIMS) Trial, which assessed 12- to 59-month-old children with recurrent moderate to severe wheezing episodes.[17] Most of the children (71%) had least 4 wheezing episodes in the past year, with 95% requiring an outpatient visit, 40% an ED visit, and 8% requiring hospitalization. Both those with and without atopic features were present in the cohort. However, those who had evidence of a higher atopy risk, as characterized by aeroallergen sensitization and positive modified asthma predictive indexes (mAPI), experienced a higher incidence of urgent care visits and hospitalizations, and oral corticosteroid (OCS) use in the prior year.

In the PEAK trial, which excluded children with significantly persistent symptoms, children treated with daily ICS had fewer symptoms and exacerbations requiring OCS during the 2-year active treatment period.[9] However, those on daily ICS were observed to have grown 0.7 cm less in height on average by the end of the trial, which seemed to be age and weight related.[18]

Given evidence of the positive effects of daily and intermittent ICS therapy in preschool children with a severe intermittent disease pattern and positive mAPI, daily low-dose and episodic high-dose ICS were compared in the Maintenance and Intermittent Inhaled Corticosteroids in Wheezing Toddlers (MIST) study.[17] Episodic high-dose ICS were started at the earliest recognized onset of respiratory tract symptoms, before progression of wheezing, for a total of 7 days. The daily low-dose ICS and episodic high-dose ICS strategies were comparable with no significant differences in asthma exacerbations or other indicators of asthma activity, control, and growth. Overall corticosteroid exposure was lower in the episodic ICS group. A 2016 metaanalysis of 5 studies and 422 participants found that episodic high-dose ICS was associated with a 35% decrease in exacerbations.[10] The number needed to treat was 6 children to prevent 1 exacerbation. This episodic ICS strategy has also been shown to decrease the use of rescue OCS.[19,20] Based on these findings, treatment for severe intermittent wheezers, particularly those with a positive mAPI, should include consideration of preemptive high-dose episodic ICS.

Although early high-dose ICS therapy can be effective in decreasing the risk of severe exacerbations among preschoolers with the severe intermittent phenotype, intermittent LTRA has not been shown to be effective. A trial of 238 children ages 12 to 58 months of age with a history of moderate to severe intermittent wheezing, composed of both positive and negative mAPI children, compared early RTI initiation of a 7-day course of budesonide, LTRA, or placebo in addition to albuterol.[17] Participants were not on concurrent controller medication. The timing of initiation was individualized, because parents received frequent education to help identify their child's symptoms that were representative of respiratory tract illness onset. Episodic treatment with budesonide or LTRA compared with placebo did not lead to a decrease in the number of episode-free days, OCS use, ED visits, hospitalizations, or quality of life. However, among the subgroup of participants with a positive mAPI status, there was evidence of decreased symptom severity during the acute illness while receiving ICS or LTRA. A subsequent metaanalysis of the efficacy of ICS and LTRA also included an analysis of this study, finding no difference in the number of the episode-free days between intermittent ICS and intermittent LTRA.[10] A 2015 Cochrane review of 4 studies of preschool children with episodic viral wheeze also found that intermittent LTRA was not associated with decreased viral episodes requiring OCS or other clinical benefits.[21]

For children with significant viral-triggered lower respiratory tract illnesses, episodic azithromycin started early in the episode is also a treatment option. Although the vast majority of lower respiratory tract illnesses are caused by viruses, bacteria are often also present and have been demonstrated to impact the risk of recurrent wheeze.[22–24] Macrolide antibiotics in particular have been studied for this purpose because of their additional antiinflammatory and antineutrophilic properties.[25,26] Two large clinical trials of the use of azithromycin early in a lower respiratory tract illness have shown efficacy in decreasing the severity or duration of the episode. The Azithromycin for Preventing the development of Upper respiratory tract Illness into Lower respiratory tract symptoms in children (APRIL) study randomized 607 children 12 to 71 months of age with a history of recurrent severe lower respiratory tract illnesses not requiring daily controller therapy.[27] The intervention was either a 5-day course of azithromycin or placebo at the earliest signs of a respiratory tract illness. Each participant was followed for 12 to 18 months and a total of 937 RTIs were treated, 80% to 83% of which had detectable virus from nasal wash samples. Azithromycin treatment was associated with a 36% decreased risk of progression to a severe episode and decreased albuterol rescue use during severe episodes. Response was independent of mAPI status and viral detection during illnesses. A randomized control trial from the Copenhagen Prospective Studies on Asthma in Childhood cohort (COPSAC) compared the use of a 3-day course of azithromycin versus placebo after at least 3 days of asthma-like episodes in 72 participants.[28] Enrolled participants had a history of recurrent asthmalike symptoms. Azithromycin use was associated with a shorter episode duration of 3.4 days, versus 7.7 days in the placebo group. Greater efficacy was seen if the therapy was started earlier in the episode, with an 83% decrease in duration when initiated before day 6 of the illness compared with a 36% decrease if started after that time.

Overall, these 2 trials provide evidence that azithromycin can mitigate lower respiratory symptoms in preschoolers with severe intermittent respiratory disease. There is concern for a risk of development of antibiotic-resistant organisms associated with repeated azithromycin treatment. In APRIL, these medications were infrequently acquired, whereas in the COPSAC cohort resistance was not assessed.[27,28] Additional research is needed.

Based on these studies, and in light of concerns regarding potential antimicrobial resistance, high-dose intermittent ICS is suggested as the preferred therapy in children with severe intermittent wheezing and evidence of atopy or sensitization. In nonatopic children, the early use of azithromycin can be considered. Because timing is crucial to its effectiveness, this treatment option should also only be reserved for a subgroup of patients whose parents have a clear understanding of the treatment plan. Monitoring for the efficacy of the response is critical.

In summary, in preschoolers with persistent asthma symptoms and evidence of atopy or allergic sensitization, a daily ICS should be trialed as the initial therapy (see **Fig. 1**). If there is no evidence of atopy or allergic sensitization, options include daily ICS, intermittent ICS, or LTRA. For the subgroup of patients with severe intermittent wheezing but who are otherwise asymptomatic between episodes, preemptive episodic high-dose ICS is effective, particularly among children with positive mAPIs. Intermittent azithromycin given early in the illness episode is also an option that decreases the risk of severe episodes, regardless of atopy status.

Based on Biomarkers

Biological markers such as blood eosinophil levels and evidence of aeroallergen sensitization have been identified as phenotypic markers predictive of treatment response. Elevated exhaled nitric oxide levels have been shown to correlate with a greater likelihood of response to ICS and can be attempted in children at least 4 years of age.[8,29] The use of pulmonary function testing is typically attempted starting at 4 to 5 years of age, owing to concerns that most children 5 years and younger cannot produce reproducible maneuvers.[8] Impulse oscillometry is another option because only tidal breathing is required (see Karen M. McDowell's article "Recent Diagnosis Techniques in Pediatric Asthma: Impulse Oscillometry in Preschool Asthma and Use of Exhaled Nitric Oxide," elsewhere in this issue). However, recent evidence supports that both impulse oscillometry and spirometry can be performed in preschool aged children; however, the literature is mixed on which method is performed more reliably and consistently in this age group.[30,31] Moreover, a recent multicenter trial of 422 children 3 to 5 year of age found that acceptable spirometry maneuvers were seen more frequently in 3-year-olds compared with 5-year-olds, suggesting that spirometry can be attempted even at 3 years of age.[32]

What to Do if First-Line Therapies Are Not Effective?

If a preschool child does not respond to first-line therapy, evaluation should include reconsideration of alternative diagnoses, assessing adherence to therapy, and reviewing inhaler and/or nebulizer techniques (**Fig. 2**). Randomized, controlled trials have shown that albuterol delivery via spacer versus nebulizer is comparable when dosing adjustments are made and treatments are administered by medical personnel in acute care settings; furthermore, no crossover trials have been performed.[33–35] There are no well-controlled trials comparing MDI and nebulization

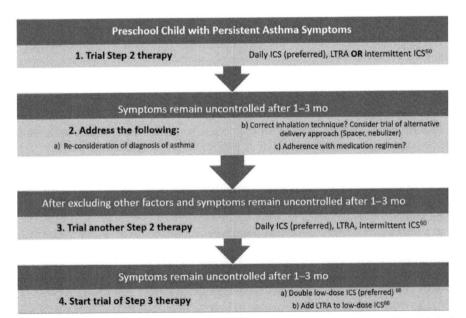

Fig. 2. Management steps for the preschool child with uncontrolled asthma. ICS, inhaled corticosteroids; LTRA, leukotriene receptor antagonist.

delivery of ICS to preschool children available. Thus, the applicability of the findings related to albuterol is uncertain when considering these delivery approaches for ICS. The decision to use a spacer versus nebulizer or switch the delivery method should be determined via assessment of the child's interaction with the delivery systems while using a shared decision-making approach with the patient's family (see **Fig. 2**).

Although significant advancements have been made in predicting response to asthma therapy, the heterogeneity of treatment response in the preschool population has not been elucidated comprehensively. If symptoms remain uncontrolled after 3 months with a given therapy, before escalating to step 3 strategies, treatment should be switched to an alternate step 2 therapy, which includes the options of daily low dose ICS, LTRA, or intermittent ICS.[8] Other step 2 therapies should be trialed before moving up to step 3 therapy, because nearly 75% of children requiring step 2 therapy exhibited a best response to at least one of these 3 strategies.[13] If step 2 therapies are still ineffective, the Global Initiative for Asthma (GINA) recommends step 3 therapies, including doubling the ICS dose or adding an LTRA to the low-dose ICS. A few trials have compared varying doses of ICS in preschool children. One randomized, controlled trial of children 6 months to 8 years old compared inhaled budesonide 0.25, 0.5, or 1.0 mg once daily versus placebo.[36] All doses improved asthma symptoms and decreased albuterol use, but only the higher 2 doses improved lung function. Another study in the same age group compared 4 inhaled budesonide regimens ranging from 0.25 mg once daily to 1.00 mg once daily.[37] All budesonide doses improved asthma control, but the lowest dose of 0.25 mg once daily was the least efficacious. The second highest dose was the only one associated with an improvement in lung function. Another trial of 4- to 8-year-old children compared 3 doses of inhaled budesonide: 0.25 mg, 0.50 mg and 1.00 mg, all given twice daily.[38] All doses improved symptoms, improved lung function, and decreased albuterol use compared with placebo, without increased adverse effects. However, no difference was found between the 3 dosing groups.

There are limited data supporting the addition of a long-acting beta agonist to the ICS in this age group. Only 1 long-acting beta agonist/ICS combination, fluticasone propionate and salmeterol, is approved in this age group, for 4 years and older.[39] However, a large safety study of 6208 children, one-third of whom were in the 4- to 6-year-old age group, demonstrated that this younger group had a comparable safety profile to the older children.[40] Studies of combination therapy with ICS and LTRA, along with moderate to high dose nonbudesonide ICS in this age group have not been performed, so this guideline recommendation is extrapolated from studies of children 6 years and older.[41]

Although anticholinergics are not currently included as a treatment option in GINA, a recent exploratory 12-week trial of 1- to 5-year-old children with uncontrolled symptoms despite ICS treatment found that the addition of tiotropium via soft mist inhaler was well-tolerated.[42] Fewer children in the tiotropium group had asthma exacerbations when compared with the placebo group, although this was an exploratory statistical analysis.

Studies of the use of biologic therapies for the treatment of asthma have not been performed in this age group. Omalizumab is the only biologic currently approved for school-age children at least 6 years of age.[43]

A key component of management is having long-term and consistent follow-up every 1 to 3 months until it is clear that adequate treatment response has been achieved.[44] Once symptoms are well-controlled, follow-up should continue to be regular, potentially every 3 to 6 months, because symptom phenotypes in this age group can evolve with time.[8,45] Step down therapy should also be considered if the child has achieved excellent asthma control for at least 3 months.

MANAGEMENT OF ACUTE EPISODES
Oral Corticosteroids

OCS are frequently prescribed for acute severe exacerbations in this age group, although there is limited evidence for consistent efficacy in this age group, and this efficacy seems to be related to severity of episode and site of care. Several studies in the preschool population have reported that OCS use in the ED setting was associated with decreased symptoms and length of hospital stay.[46–48] A multicenter trial of children ages 1 to 17 years with moderate or severe asthma receiving OCS and inhaled bronchodilators in the ED found that OCS dosing was not associated with management failure, defined as subsequent hospitalization, prolonged symptoms, and rebound ED visits.[49]

A large randomized, controlled trial in 2009 by Panickar and colleagues[50] assessed 700 patients ages 10 to 60 months of age who had mild to moderate wheezing associated with viral infections evaluated in an ED setting who were subsequently hospitalized. Approximately 35% were first time wheezers. A 5-day prednisolone course was compared with placebo, and no decreases in duration of hospital stay, albuterol use or 7-day symptom scores were found. Potential confounders of the negative findings include the likely inclusion of bronchiolitis in a substantial proportion of patients, a condition for which OCS are known to be an ineffective therapy, because children as young as 10 months of age with first-time wheezing were included in the study.[51]

A subsequent large, single-center, randomized trial by Foster and colleagues[52] included older children, between 2 and 5 years of age, to help minimize the inclusion of bronchiolitis episodes during the study. Enrolled children had virus-associated wheezing presenting to the ED and were randomized to 3 days of prednisolone 1 mg/kg/d or placebo. A virus was identified in two-thirds of the participants. Compared with the Panickar and colleagues[51] study, these participants had more severe wheezing per pulmonary score. Approximately two-thirds of the prednisolone and placebo groups were subsequently admitted. The primary outcome was the total length of hospital stay and was found to be 170 minutes shorter in the prednisolone-treated group. The total time was 6.2 hours versus 9.0 hours in the prednisolone and placebo groups, respectively. It is possible that the prednisolone-treated patients may have been able to avoid hospitalization altogether, but this could not be assessed because the ED had a 4-hour maximum observation time requirement to maximize room availability.[53] As part of a post hoc analysis, a hospital length of stay greater than 12 hours occurred in 25% in the prednisolone treated group compared with 38% in the placebo group, a 34% decrease.[52] A limitation of this study is that it was a single-center study. Furthermore, it was initially intended to be a noninferiority analysis, then changed post hoc to a superiority analysis, although this was done before the analysis began. Overall, these findings suggest that the initiation of OCS in the ED may decrease the duration of hospitalization, with the potential to avoid admission altogether.

In contrast with its use in the ED and inpatient setting, research supporting parent-initiated, outpatient use of OCS for acute exacerbations remains weak.[8] Most of the studies have not detected an improvement in symptom scores or rate of ED/hospitalization visits.[54–57] Additionally, unfavorable associations have been noted in a few studies, including an increased rate of hospitalization in 1 study, and an increased number of outpatient visits in another study.[55,56] These findings may be related to prednisone-associated behavioral changes. It is possible that OCS efficacy in this outpatient setting has not been demonstrated because prior studies had variable study designs, were often underpowered, and most outpatient episodes are relatively mild in severity and demonstrate rapid and spontaneous resolution, such that an accelerated resolution with OCS may not be possible.[54]

Specific subgroups that may derive benefit from outpatient OCS use have not been identified yet. In particular, those with evidence of atopic sensitization might be thought to be possible candidates because they are known to respond to ICS and are more likely to continue having persistent asthma.[57] A post hoc analysis of the AIMS and Maintenance and Intermittent Inhaled Corticosteroids in Wheezing Toddlers (MIST) trials found that outpatient episodes treated with OCS did not resolve more rapidly when treated with OCS relative to episodes of comparable severity not managed with OCS.[54] The majority of patients in these 2 trials (60% of the AIMS patients and all MIST participants) had a positive mAPI. Furthermore, Oommen and colleagues[55] stratified 1- to 5-year-old children by high or low serum eosinophil cation protein and eosinophilic protein X, which is not a included component of the mAPI but may potentially be a surrogate marker. No symptom improvement from parent-initiated systemic corticosteroid use was found.

In summary, additional research regarding the role of OCS in treating preschool asthma exacerbations is needed, particularly studies focusing on specific subgroups that may respond more favorably, such as those with evidence of atopic predisposition or sensitization. In the meantime, OCS remain as a therapeutic option for more severe episodes, but should be used judiciously.[8] Maximal home albuterol use should be applied as a first-line treatment and, if systemic corticosteroids are prescribed, treatment duration should be minimized, and side effects should be monitored closely.

MANAGEMENT OF LIMITING FACTORS
Provider Related

Other differential diagnoses can masquerade as asthma in this age group and need to remain under consideration. These diagnoses include bronchiolitis, structural abnormalities such as right-sided aortic arch or vascular sling, chronic lung disease, foreign body disease, and cystic fibrosis, and are reviewed elsewhere.[58]

Barriers to Adherence

There are multiple potential barriers to treatment adherence in this age group, which should be considered when monitoring a preschool child with uncontrolled asthma symptoms. Owing to their age-appropriate but limited ability to perceive and communicate asthma symptoms, their parents have the challenging role of identifying and monitoring signs of asthma. Administering daily medication, particularly nonpill medications such as ICS, which require somewhat prolonged cooperation from the child, can be difficult to achieve especially because many parents rely on multiple caregivers for their children.[59] Parental concern for side effects or manifestations of side effects associated with daily medication can also affect adherence. High medication cost, depending on the family's insurance status, can also be a barrier. Additionally, when a child is on multiple medications with different prescribed schedules, the complexity can increase the likelihood of nonadherence. The delivery system can also affect adherence, because individual children may better tolerate a spacer over a nebulizer, or vice versa. Improper technique can also be a barrier to adequate medication intake, and technique should be reviewed on a fairly regular basis as needed, particularly if symptoms are uncontrolled. Consideration of these factors is essential in developing a personalized and effective treatment plan.

Side Effects

Decreases in growth velocity have been reported with ICS use. Results from the PEAK study showed that, in the preschool population, low-dose daily ICS was associated with less linear growth in those of younger age and lower weight.[18] Although there is some evidence for the safety and tolerability of medium or high dose ICS use, research of potential long term effects such as impaired linear growth is needed.[37,60] OCS burst use is known to be associated with decreases in linear growth, although the degree of risk associated with each additional OCS course remains to be characterized. Characterizing the effects of behavioral changes related to OCS use is also needed.[55,56] Thus, the monitoring of growth is an essential component of care for preschool children with asthma.

SUMMARY AND FUTURE DIRECTIONS

Preschool asthma is a heterogeneous condition that can change over time. Recent studies have begun to crystallize evidence-based and phenotype-directed approaches for the young child with recurrent wheezing and asthma and can help predict treatment response. Clinical judgment and regular reevaluation remain essential in devising an optimal individualized treatment plan for each patient.

More research is needed to better understand the therapeutic options beyond step 2 GINA recommendations in this population.[8] Some data are available for high-dose budesonide.[36–38,44] Additional studies of ICS in combination with long-acting beta agonist, LTRA, and/or tiotropium, along with moderate to high doses of nonbudesonide ICS in this age group, are needed. No biologic studies have been conducted in children, but may represent an opportunity for early treatment and prevention in preschool children with significant atopic disease.

REFERENCES

1. Akinbami LJ, Moorman JE, Garbe PL, et al. Status of childhood asthma in the United States, 1980–2007. Pediatrics 2009;123(Supplement 3):S131–45.
2. Martinez FD, Wright AL, Taussig LM, et al. Asthma and wheezing in the first six years of life. N Engl J Med 1995;332(3):133–8.
3. Ly NP, Gold DR, Weiss ST, et al. Recurrent wheeze in early childhood and asthma among children at risk for atopy. Pediatrics 2006;117(6):e1132–8.
4. Bacharier LB. The recurrently wheezing preschool child - Benign or asthma in the making? Ann Allergy Asthma Immunol 2015;115(6):463–70.
5. Castro-Rodriguez J, Holberg CJ, Wright AL, et al. A clinical index to define risk of asthma in young children with recurrent wheezing. Am J Respir Crit Care Med 2000;162(4):1403–6.
6. Guilbert TW, Morgan WJ, Krawiec M, et al. The prevention of early asthma in kids study: design, rationale and methods for the childhood asthma research and education network. Control Clin Trials 2004;25(3):286–310.
7. Chang TS, Lemanske RF, Guilbert TW, et al. Evaluation of the modified asthma predictive index in high-risk preschool children. J Allergy Clin Immunol Pract 2013;1(2):152–6.
8. Global Initiative for Asthma. Global Strategy for Asthma Management and Prevention, 2018. Available at: https://ginasthma.org/2018-gina-report-global-strategy-for-asthma-management-and-prevention.

9. Guilbert TW, Morgan WJ. Long-term inhaled corticosteroids in preschool children at high risk for asthma. N Engl J Med 2006;354(19):1985–97.

10. Kaiser SV, Huynh T, Bacharier LB, et al. Preventing exacerbations in preschoolers with recurrent wheeze: a meta-analysis. Pediatrics 2016;137(6):e20154496.

11. Castro-Rodriguez JA, Rodrigo GJ. Efficacy of inhaled corticosteroids in infants and preschoolers with recurrent wheezing and asthma: a systematic review with meta-analysis. Pediatrics 2009;123(3):e519–25.

12. Bacharier LB, Guilbert TW, Zeiger RS, et al. Patient characteristics associated with improved outcomes with use of an inhaled corticosteroid in preschool children at risk for asthma. J Allergy Clin Immunol 2009;123(5). https://doi.org/10.1016/j.jaci.2008.12.1120.

13. Fitzpatrick AM, Jackson DJ, Mauger DT, et al. Individualized therapy for persistent asthma in young children. J Allergy Clin Immunol 2016;138(6):1608–18.e12.

14. Bacharier LB, Phillips BR, Bloomberg GR, et al. Severe intermittent wheezing in preschool children: a distinct phenotype. J Allergy Clin Immunol 2007;119(3):604–10.

15. Beigelman A, Bacharier LB. Management of preschool children with recurrent wheezing: lessons from the NHLBI's asthma research networks. J Allergy Clin Immunol Pract 2016;4(1):1–8.

16. Spycher BD, Silverman M, Pescatore AM, et al. Comparison of phenotypes of childhood wheeze and cough in 2 independent cohorts. J Allergy Clin Immunol 2013;132(5):1058–67.

17. Bacharier LB, Phillips BR, Zeiger RS, et al. Episodic use of an inhaled corticosteroid or leukotriene receptor antagonist in preschool children with moderate-to-severe intermittent wheezing. J Allergy Clin Immunol 2008;122(6):1127–43.

18. Guilbert TW, Mauger DT, Allen DB, et al. Growth of preschool children at high risk for asthma 2 years after discontinuation of fluticasone. J Allergy Clin Immunol 2011;128(5). https://doi.org/10.1016/j.jaci.2011.06.027.

19. Ducharme FM, Lemire C, Noya FJD, et al. Preemptive use of high-dose fluticasone for virus-induced wheezing in young children. N Engl J Med 2009;360(4):339–53. https://doi.org/10.1542/peds.2009-1870RRR.

20. McKean M, Ducharme F. Inhaled steroids for episodic viral wheeze of childhood. Cochrane Database Syst Rev 2000;(2):CD001107.

21. Brodlie M, Gupta A, Rodriguez-Martinez CE, et al. Leukotriene receptor antagonists as maintenance and intermittent therapy for episodic viral wheeze in children. Cochrane Database Syst Rev 2015;2015(10). https://doi.org/10.1002/14651858.CD008202.pub2.

22. Zhou Y, Bacharier L, Isaacson-Schmid M, et al. Azithromycin therapy during respiratory syncytial virus bronchiolitis : upper airway microbiome alterations and subsequent recurrent wheeze. J Allergy Clin Immunol 2016;138(4):1215–9.e5.

23. Suárez-Arrabal MC, Mella C, Lopez SM, et al. Nasopharyngeal bacterial burden and antibiotics: influence on inflammatory markers and disease severity in infants with respiratory syncytial virus bronchiolitis. J Infect 2015;71(4):458–69.

24. Carlsson CJ, Vissing NH, Sevelsted A, et al. Duration of wheezy episodes in early childhood is independent of the microbial trigger. J Allergy Clin Immunol 2015;136(5):1208–14.

25. Simpson JL, Powell H, Boyle MJ, et al. Clarithromycin targets neutrophilic airway inflammation in refractory asthma. Am J Respir Crit Care Med 2008;177(2):148–55.

26. Cameron EJ, Mcsharry C, Chaudhuri R, et al. Long-term macrolide treatment of chronic inflammatory airway diseases: risks, benefits and future developments. Clin Exp Allergy 2012;42(9):1302–12.

27. Bacharier LB, Guilbert TW, Mauger DT, et al. Early Administration of azithromycin and prevention of severe lower respiratory tract illnesses in preschool children with a history of such illnesses a randomized clinical trial. JAMA 2015;314(19): 2034–44.

28. Stokholm J, Chawes BL, Vissing NH, et al. Azithromycin for episodes with asthma-like symptoms in young children aged 1-3 years: a randomised, double-blind, placebo-controlled trial. Lancet Respir Med 2016;4(1):19–26.

29. Burbank A, Szefler S. Current and future management of the young child with early onset wheezing. Curr Opin Allergy Clin Immunol 2017;17(2):146–52.

30. Komarow HD, Myles IA, Uzzaman A, et al. Impulse oscillometry in the evaluation of diseases of the airways in children. Ann Allergy Asthma Immunol 2011;106:191–9.

31. Goldman MD. Clinical application of forced oscillation. Pulm Pharmacol Ther 2001;14:341–50.

32. Kattan M, Bacharier LB, O'Connor GT, et al. Spirometry and impulse oscillometry in preschool children: acceptability and relationship to maternal smoking in pregnancy. J Allergy Clin Immunol Pract 2018. https://doi.org/10.1016/j.jaip.2017.12. 028.

33. Cates CJ, Rowe BH, Bara A. Holding chambers (spacers) versus nebulisers for beta-agonist treatment of acute asthma. Cochrane Database Syst Rev 2013;(9):CD000052.

34. Mitselou N, Hedlin G, Hederos CA. Spacers versus nebulizers in treatment of acute asthma – a prospective randomized study in preschool children. J Asthma 2016;53(10):1059–62.

35. Ploin D, Chapuis FR, Stamm D, et al. High-dose albuterol by metered-dose inhaler plus a spacer device versus nebulization in preschool children with recurrent wheezing: a double-blind, randomized equivalence trial. Pediatrics 2000; 106(2 Pt 1):311–7.

36. Kemp JP, Skoner DP, Szefler SJ, et al. Once-daily budesonide inhalation suspension for the treatment of persistent asthma in infants and young children. Ann Allergy Asthma Immunol 1999;83(3):231–9.

37. Baker JW, Mellon M, Wald J, et al. A multiple-dosing, placebo-controlled study of budesonide inhalation suspension given once or twice daily for treatment of persistent asthma in young children and infants. Pediatrics 1999;103(2): 414–21.

38. Shapiro G, Mendelson L, Kraemer MJ, et al. Efficacy and safety of budesonide inhalation suspension (pulmicort respules) in young children with inhaled steroid-dependent, persistent asthma. J Allergy Clin Immunol 1998;102(5): 789–96.

39. GlaxoSmithKline. Advair diskus prescribing information. 2017. Available at: https://www.gsksource.com/pharma/content/dam/GlaxoSmithKline/US/en/Prescribing_Information/Advair_Diskus/pdf/ADVAIR-DISKUS-PI-PIL-IFU.PDF. Accessed June 1, 2018.

40. Stempel DA, Szefler SJ, Pedersen S, et al. Safety of adding salmeterol to fluticasone propionate in children with asthma. N Engl J Med 2016;375(9):840–9.

41. Lemanske RF, Mauger DT, Sorkness CA, et al. Step-up therapy for children with uncontrolled asthma receiving inhaled corticosteroids. N Engl J Med 2010; 362(11):975–85.

42. Vrijlandt EJLE, El Azzi G, Vandewalker M, et al. Safety and efficacy of tiotropium in children aged 1–5 years with persistent asthmatic symptoms: a randomised, double-blind, placebo-controlled trial. Lancet Respir Med 2018;6(2):127–37.
43. Full prescribing information, XOLAIR. New Jersey: Xolair Website, Genentech USA, Inc; 2018.
44. Chipps BE, Bacharier LB, Farrar JR, et al. The pediatric asthma yardstick: practical recommendations for a sustained step-up in asthma therapy for children with inadequately controlled asthma. Ann Allergy Asthma Immunol 2018;120(6): 559–79.e11.
45. Pedersen SE, Hurd SS, Lemanske RF, et al. Global strategy for the diagnosis and management of asthma in children 5 years and younger. Pediatr Pulmonol 2011; 46(1):1–17.
46. Tal A, Levy N, Bearman J. Methylprednisolone therapy for acute asthma in infants and toddlers: a controlled clinical trial. Pediatrics 1990;86(3):350–6. Available at: http://pediatrics.aappublications.org/content/86/3/350.short.
47. Csonka P, Kaila M, Laippala P, et al. Oral prednisolone in the acute management of children age 6 to 35 months with viral respiratory infection-induced lower airway disease: a randomized, placebo-controlled trial. J Pediatr 2003;143(03): 725–30.
48. Jartti T, Nieminen R, Vuorinen T, et al. Short- and long-term efficacy of prednisolone for first acute rhinovirus-induced wheezing episode. J Allergy Clin Immunol 2015;135(3):691–8.e9.
49. Ducharme FM, Zemek R, Chauhan BF, et al. Factors associated with failure of emergency department management in children with acute moderate or severe asthma: a prospective, multicentre, cohort study. Lancet Respir Med 2016; 4(12):990–8.
50. Panickar J, Lakhanpaul M, Lambert PC, et al. Oral prednisolone for preschool children with acute virus-induced wheezing. N Engl J Med 2009;360(4):329–38.
51. Corneli HM, Zorc JJ, Mahajan P, et al. A multicenter, randomized, controlled trial of dexamethasone for bronchiolitis. N Engl J Med 2007;357(4):331–9.
52. Foster SJ, Cooper MN, Oosterhof S, et al. Oral prednisolone in preschool children with virus-associated wheeze: a prospective, randomised, double-blind, placebo-controlled trial. Lancet Respir Med 2018;97–106. https://doi.org/10.1016/S2213-2600(18)30008-0.
53. Zorc JJ. Oral corticosteroids reduce length of hospital stay for preschool children with virus-associated wheeze. Lancet Respir Med 2018;6:76–7.
54. Beigelman A, King TS, Mauger D, et al. Do oral corticosteroids reduce the severity of acute lower respiratory tract illnesses in preschool children with recurrent wheezing? J Allergy Clin Immunol 2013;131(6):1518–25.e14.
55. Oommen A, Lambert PC, Grigg J. Efficacy of a short course of parent-initiated oral prednisolone for viral wheeze in children aged 1-5 years: randomised controlled trial. Lancet 2003;362(9394):1433–8.
56. Grant CC, Duggan AK, DeAngelis C. Independent parental administration of prednisone in acute asthma: a double-blind, placebo-controlled, crossover study. Pediatrics 1995;96(2):224–9. Available at: http://www.ncbi.nlm.nih.gov/pubmed/7630674.
57. Beigelman A, Durrani S, Guilbert TW. Should a preschool child with acute episodic wheeze be treated with oral corticosteroids? A pro/con debate. J Allergy Clin Immunol Pract 2016;4(1):27–35.
58. Strunk RC. Defining asthma in the preschool-aged child. Pediatrics 2002;109(2 Suppl):357–61.

59. Rand CS. Adherence to asthma therapy in the preschool child. Allergy 2002;57: 48–57.

60. Bisgaard H, Gillies J, Groenewald M, et al, Maden C on behalf of an ISG. The effect of inhaled fluticasone propionate in the treatment of young asthmatic children: a dose comparison study. Am J Respir Crit Care Med 1999;160(9): 126–31.

Management/Comorbidities of School-Aged Children with Asthma

Carolyn M. Kercsmar, MD[a],*, Cassie Shipp, MD[b]

KEYWORDS

- Asthma • Pediatric • Management • Comorbidities

KEY POINTS

- Asthma in early childhood is a heterogeneous disease, with the classification moving toward a more phenotypic approach.
- Asthma management encompasses treatment of the disease itself as well as the management of comorbidities and education of patient and family.
- Untreated comorbidities may result in poor asthma control. It is important to treat comorbidities before escalation of asthma therapies.

INTRODUCTION

Asthma is a disorder characterized by intermittent, reversible airflow obstruction that occurs as a result of dysregulated airway epithelial function and inflammation. This obstruction may resolve spontaneously or may resolve only after medical treatment. An estimated 7 million children younger than 18 have asthma in the United States.[1] An accurate diagnosis is important and is supported by the addition of objective measurement of airflow obstruction and/or hyperreactivity with pulmonary function testing in school-aged children. Effective asthma management in this age group should address 3 broad domains: pharmacologic treatment, treatment of comorbid conditions, and patient and caregiver education.

MANAGEMENT OF ASTHMA

Although the diagnosis of asthma is defined by reversible airway obstruction, it is becoming clear that this term encompasses several very different phenotypes. These

Disclosure Statement: No financial or commercial disclosures.
[a] Department of Pediatrics, University of Cincinnati College of Medicine, Division of pulmonary Medicine, Cincinnati Children's Hospital Medical Center, Cincinnati Children's Hospital, 3333 Burnet Avenue, MLC 7041, Cincinnati, OH 45229, USA; [b] Division of Pulmonary Medicine, Cincinnati Children's Hospital Medical Center, Cincinnati Children's Hospital, 3333 Burnet Avenue, MLC 7041, Cincinnati, OH 45229, USA
* Corresponding author.
E-mail address: Carolyn.kercsmar@cchmc.org

Immunol Allergy Clin N Am 39 (2019) 191–204
https://doi.org/10.1016/j.iac.2018.12.004
0889-8561/19/© 2018 Elsevier Inc. All rights reserved.

distinct phenotypes may have different underlying pathophysiology (endotypes), different natural history, different genetic basis, and, most important to the clinician, different response to treatment. As the understanding of the phenotypic differences in pediatric asthma continues to increase, the pharmacologic and clinical management strategies will also evolve (see Nathan M. Pajor and Theresa W. Guilbert's article, "Personalized Medicine and Pediatric Asthma," in this issue). Although still evolving, there are several identifiable pediatric asthma phenotypes present in school-aged children. The most common phenotype is the allergic. These children typically present with eczema early in life, allergic sensitization, and recurrent wheeze. The airway inflammation and reactivity appear to be mediated by Th2 cytokines, along with related biomarkers, including elevated eosinophils, elevated immunoglobulin E (IgE), and/or elevated exhaled nitric oxide.[2] A smaller subset of school-aged children is nonallergic and exhibits primarily neutrophilic airway inflammation. Treatment targeted at neutrophilic inflammation may be of more benefit for these patients.[3] There is also crossover between the 2 phenotypes, with some patients presenting with both neutrophilic and allergic-mediated inflammation. Occasionally there is no predominant airway inflammatory cellular pattern (paucicellular). Similar to the preschool pediatric population, school-aged children may continue to experience primarily viral triggered asthma, with very few symptoms outside of illness. Exercise-induced bronchospasm (EIB), with or without underlying chronic asthma, may also present in the school-aged child. The pathophysiology that underlies EIB has been hypothesized to be different than the previously discussed asthma phenotypes, with mast cell degranulation triggered by change in osmolar environment or vascular changes brought on by exercise.[4]

Currently there are several accepted strategies for managing pediatric asthma in the school-aged child. The stepwise approach to childhood asthma management, as described by the National Heart, Lung, and Blood Institute and Global Initiative for Asthma (GINA) guidelines, recommends initial grading of severity and/or control based on individual assessment of impairment and risk.[5,6] Impairment focuses on daily symptom burden (wheeze/cough, nocturnal awakenings, daily short-acting beta-agonist use, and activity limitations) and lung function. Risk refers to past and future exacerbations requiring medical attention and/or the use of systemic steroids as well as risk of loss of lung function over time, poor airway growth, and medication adverse effect. Although the combined assessment of impairment and risk allows for stratification of disease severity in the treatment-naive child, the emphasis on a priori severity classification is currently viewed as less important than achieving and maintaining good control. After treatment, it is possible to classify asthma into intermittent mild, moderate, and severe persistent categories based on level of treatment necessary to achieve control.

Pharmacologic strategies for asthma (discussed in more detail later) are based on degree of control and frequency/severity of exacerbations in the previous year. For patients with very infrequent symptoms and low exacerbation risk (intermittent asthma), short-acting beta-agonist therapy (SABA) is recommended on an as-needed basis, with acute exacerbation management with systemic steroids. If patients require frequent SABA use or have more than one exacerbation per year, therapy is escalated. Mild, moderate, and severe persistent asthma share the need for daily controller therapy, with the most common and effective being inhaled corticosteroids (ICS). The dosing of ICS as well as when to combine with additional therapy, such as a leukotriene receptor antagonist (LTRA) or long-acting beta-agonist (LABA), is adjusted based on the patient response to therapy. It is important to frequently reassess asthma control to determine the need for adjustment in step therapy[5,6] (**Figs. 1** and **2**).

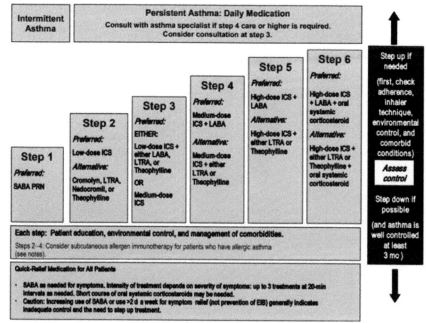

Notes:

- The stepwise approach is meant to assist, not replace, the clinical decisionmaking required to meet individual patient needs.

- If alternative treatment is used and response is inadequate, discontinue it and use the preferred treatment before stepping up.

- Theophylline is a less desirable alternative due to the need to monitor serum concentration levels.

- Step 1 and step 2 medications are based on Evidence A. Step 3 ICS + adjunctive therapy and ICS are based on Evidence B for efficacy of each treatment and extrapolation from comparator trials in older children and adults—comparator trials are not available for this age group; steps 4–6 are based on expert opinion and extrapolation from studies in older children and adults.

- Immunotherapy for steps 2–4 is based on Evidence B for house-dust mites, animal danders, and pollens; evidence is weak or lacking for molds and cockroaches. Evidence is strongest for immunotherapy with single allergens. The role of allergy in asthma is greater in children than in adults. Clinicians who administer immunotherapy should be prepared and equipped to identify and treat anaphylaxis that may occur.

Fig. 1. The stepwise approach for management of asthma in children aged 5 to 11. PRN, as needed. (*From* National Heart, Lung, and Blood Institute (NHLBI). Expert panel report 3: guidelines for the diagnosis and management of asthma. 2007. Available at: https://www.nhlbi.nih.gov/health-topics/guidelines-for-diagnosis-management-of-asthma. Accessed October 10, 2018; with permission.)

There are several validated tools to aid in assessing asthma control in children, and use of these tools is endorsed by guideline statements.[7,8] The Childhood Asthma Control Test and the Asthma Control Questionnaire are the most commonly used in the school-aged population.[7] These questionnaires obtain responses from the patient and family regarding symptom frequency, activity limitation, SABA use, and global well-being. Recall bias and underrecognition of symptoms may affect scoring of the questionnaire; however, they still remain an important part of regular assessment of asthma control.

PHARMACOLOGIC TREATMENT
Intermittent Asthma

Children with intermittent asthma or EIB have brief, infrequent wheeze or cough that is easily relieved with inhaled SABA treatment and occur no more frequently than once or

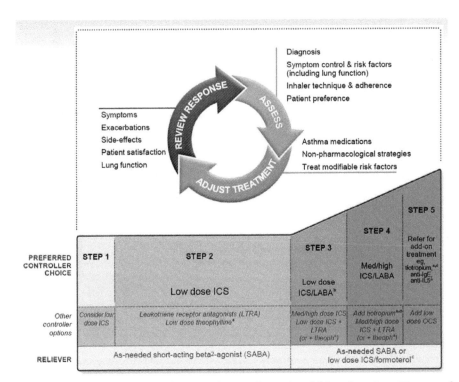

Fig. 2. Stepwise management: pharmacotherapy. [a] Not for children less than 12 years of age. [b] For children 6 to 11 years old, the preferred step 3 treatment is medium-dose ICS. [c] For patients prescribed BDP/formoterol or BUD/formoterol maintenance and reliever therapy. [d] Tiotropium by mist inhaler is an add-on treatment for patients ≥12 years of age with a history of exacerbations. IL5, interleukin 5; theoph, theophylline. (*From* Global Initiative for Asthma. Global strategy for asthma management and prevention. 2018. Available at: www.ginasthma.org/. Accessed October 18, 2018; with permission.)

twice per week. However, the most recent GINA guidelines suggest that use of as-needed SABA as sole asthma treatment be restricted to those with mild symptoms that occur no more often than once or twice per month and that the patients have no risk factors for exacerbations.[5] Treatment is with inhaled SABA at a dose of 2 to 6 puffs (albuterol, 90 µg/puff) every 3 to 4 hours or 0.15 mg/kg (usual dose 2.5 mg, maximum 5 mg) nebulized from a small-volume nebulizer. Numerous studies have demonstrated that administration of albuterol by MDI is equally effective as that given by nebulizer. Moreover, metered dose inhaler (MDI) use (with or without a valved holding chamber) is more convenient and less expensive than a nebulizer. EIB largely may be prevented with inhalation of albuterol (or formoterol) 5 to 20 minutes before exercise. Montelukast taken 1 to 2 hours before exercise may also help prevent EIB.

Mild Persistent Asthma

Most young children with asthma have mild persistent disease, based on symptoms that occur several times per week, but not daily, infrequent nocturnal symptoms, and normal pulmonary function. Exacerbations that require medical treatment occur once or twice per year. Preferred treatment of mild persistent asthma with an allergic or T2-high phenotype (elevated fractional exhaled nitric oxide, peripheral eosinophilia, elevated allergen-specific IgE, or positive skin tests) is low-dose ICS. Evidence strongly supports the efficacy of ICS compared with other treatments in improving pulmonary function, reducing symptoms, exacerbations, and bronchial hyperreactivity. The safety profile for ICS given at low dose is excellent for most children. Few data suggest that one type of ICS offers significantly greater benefit than others, and the dose equivalency differs (**Table 1**).

Beclomethasone, fluticasone, and budesonide have been extensively studied in children, are available in multiple devices (MDI, DPI, SVN), and are well tolerated by most patients, and the adverse event profile is well understood. There are few large comparative effectiveness trials in children. One retrospective observational study comparing BDP to FP found a slight advantage in reducing exacerbations for BDP, but may have missed symptom control differences that were not assessed.[9] Newer inhaled steroids, such as mometasone, fluticasone furoate, and ciclesonide, have comparable efficacy to BDP and FP; these newer preparations are effective at once-a-day dosing for many patients.

Chronic daily administration of ICS is the standard recommendation to maintain good asthma control in children with mild asthma, but recent data support intermittent dosing strategies for some patients. This strategy appears to benefit the risk domain more than the impairment domain; therefore, if daily symptom burden reduction is more important than mild exacerbation reduction, a daily treatment strategy may be preferable.[10]

A study comparing daily with as-needed use of BDP in children with mild asthma who were previously well controlled while taking daily low-dose ICS showed that those who received BDP daily (40 μg twice a day) and as a rescue (with albuterol) or as rescue only (80 μg with each 2 puffs of albuterol) had fewer exacerbations than the placebo group. However, only the daily BDP group had a significant risk reduction, but the results did not reach statistical significance (exacerbation probability 31% for BDP daily; 35% for BDP as rescue only, $P = .07$; 49% for placebo with albuterol rescue). However, linear growth was more than 1 cm lower in both groups who received inhaled steroids daily compared with placebo ($P<.0001$), and no significant difference in growth between the placebo group and those who received BDP only as a rescue medication. These data suggest that some patients with mild asthma may have fewer exacerbations with intermittent ICS use and less risk of growth suppression. However, daily use of low-dose ICS provides the best overall control.[11]

An alternative treatment of mild asthma is an LTRA, such as montelukast, with once-a-day oral administration and only uncommon mild adverse effects (ie, nausea, headache, vivid dreams). Although the current National Asthma Education and Prevention Program guidelines still list cromolyn and theophylline as alternative treatments, cromolyn has limited efficacy and availability and theophylline has complicated dosing and monitoring requirements.

For patients who are not responsive to ICS or LTRA, particularly those with a neutrophilic or nonatopic phenotype, treatment with macrolide antibiotics (largely azithromycin) has been explored. There have been a few small studies in children that demonstrate improvement in symptom-free days as well as a decrease in acute episode duration and reduction in airway reactivity with azithromycin.[12] In addition, a large double-blind placebo-controlled trial in young children showed that a 5-day course of azithromycin administered at the onset of an upper respiratory tract infection in children 1 to 6 years of age resulted in significantly fewer episodes of severe wheezing-associated episodes compared with placebo.[13] Further studies are needed to determine the efficacy of and patient phenotype responsive to macrolide treatment of asthma.

Table 1
Estimated comparative daily doses for inhaled corticosteroids

Drug	Low Daily Dose	Medium Daily Dose	High Daily Dose
Beclomethasone HFA 40 or 80 µg/puff	80–160 µg	>160–320 µg	>320 µg
Budesonide Suspension for nebulization dry powder (90, 180, or 200 µg/inhalation)	0.5 mg 180–400 µg	1.0 mg 400–800 µg	>2.0 mg >800 µg
Fluticasone dipropionate HFA/MDI: 44, 110, 220 µg/puff	88–176 µg	>176–352 µg	>352 µg
DPI: 50, 100, 250 µg/puff	100–200 µg	200–400 µg	>400 µg
Fluticasone furoate 100, 200 µg/puff	NA	NA	NA
Mometasone DPI 110, 220 µg/puff	110 µg	110–220 µg	>400 µg
MDI, 100, 200 µg/puff	100 µg	100–200 µg	>400 µg
Ciclesonide MDI 80, 160 µg/puff	NA	NA	NA

Abbreviations: BDP, beclomethasone dipropionate; DPI, dry powder inhaler; FP, fluticasone propionate; HFA, hydrofluoroalkane; MDI, metered dose inhaler; NA, not approved for this age group; SVN, small volume nebulizer.

Adapted from National Heart, Lung, and Blood Institute (NHLBI). Expert panel report 3: guidelines for the diagnosis and management of asthma. 2007. Available at: https://www.nhlbi.nih.gov/health-topics/guidelines-for-diagnosis-management-of-asthma. Accessed October 11, 2018; with permission.

Children who have frequent symptoms and/or exacerbations while being treated with low-dose ICSs have moderate disease, and their treatment should be stepped up. Current recommendations include increasing the ICS dose to the moderate range or adding a second controller drug and continuing low-dose ICS. Although the dose response curve for ICS plateaus at relatively modest doses, some patients may derive further improvement in symptom control and exacerbation reduction with higher daily ICS amounts. Patients treated with ICS beyond the low range should be closely monitored because the risk of growth suppression is raised. Failure to achieve improved control after a 3-month trial should prompt a change in strategy. A multicenter, double-blind randomized triple-crossover study using a composite of 3 outcomes (exacerbations, asthma-control days, and forced expiratory volume in 1 second [FEV_1]) demonstrated a differential response to the treatment steps (moderate-dose ICS, low-dose ICS plus LABA, low-dose ICS + LTRA) in 161 of the 165 children enrolled.[14] The response to LABA step-up was the best option compared with LTRA or increasing the ICS dose. White race or Hispanic ethnicity predicted a better response to LABA; African Americans were as likely to respond to LABA as to ICS step-up therapy and least likely to respond to LTRA. The effect of all step-up options was on symptom control, but none of the options reduced acute asthma exacerbations. Because this trial was relatively short (16 weeks), long-term maintenance of effect remains uncertain.

LABAs are the current add-on drugs of choice, and substantial evidence indicates efficacy and effectiveness.[15,16] Fixed-dose combinations of fluticasone and salmeterol, budesonide, or mometasone and formoterol, and more recently, fluticasone furoate plus vilanterol in a single inhaler make this treatment modality attractive. A recent large randomized controlled trial demonstrated the safety of the ICS + LABA combination in children with asthma as compared with ICS alone.[17] Children treated for 6 months with ICS + LABA had fewer, albeit not statistically significant, serious exacerbations than those treated with ICS alone at equivalent doses. Importantly, there was no safety signal with addition of LABA in the form of asthma hospitalizations, intubations, or deaths. Although the additive effect of LTRA, such as montelukast, to low- or medium-dose ICS is more limited, it can be effective for some patients.

Another strategy to treat inadequate or loss of control in patients who continue to experience symptoms or exacerbations while being treated with low-dose ICS is the intermittent use of an ICS + LABA. This paradigm requires the use of ICS like mometasone or budesonide plus formoterol as both rescue and controller medication.[18] The ICS + LABA is administered in place of SABA when experiencing symptoms. Budesonide/formoterol used as needed prolonged the time to the first and subsequent severe exacerbations, resulting in more than 40% lower exacerbation risk compared with daily higher-dose ICS treatment plus SABA. This as-needed regimen also reduced severe exacerbation rates, improved symptoms, awakenings, and lung function compared with fixed-dosing regimens.[19,20] The timing of the administration of the ICS (at first sign of symptoms) along with the LABA is likely a key factor in improving outcomes. Data on the use of this intermittent strategy to manage asthma in school-aged children remain limited.

To avoid loss of asthma control progressing to an exacerbation, increasing the dose of ICS temporarily, usually at the first sign of an upper respiratory tract infection or acute increase in symptoms, has been attempted. Doubling the prescribed daily dose of ICS has been shown to be ineffective, but there have been reports of effectiveness of quadruple doses. A recently published randomized controlled trial of quintupling the dose of ICS (from 176 μg/d fluticasone to 880 μg/d) for 7 days in children aged 5 to 11 years with mild-moderate asthma, demonstrated no significant reduction in exacerbations with the high-dose ICS.[21] Children in the high-dose group had significantly higher ICS exposure over 12 months and a reduction in growth rate. Although high-dose ICS to prevent exacerbations may work in some populations, there is concern that it may not be effective for school-aged children.

LTRA when added to inhaled BUD in one study resulted in a modest improvement in peak expiratory flow rate (PEFR) and a reduction in need for SABA.[22] Low-dose theophylline is another add-on medication that may also improve symptom control. A single daily dose of theophylline time-release preparation can be well tolerated and is typically less expensive than using an LABA or LTRA. However, drug-drug interactions can be significant. Tiotropium, a long-acting muscarinic receptor antagonist with a duration of action of 24 hours, has recently been approved for use in children aged 6 years in the United States and added as recommended therapy for children aged ≥12 years in steps 4 and 5 of the most recent version of the GINA guidelines.[5] Tiotropium has high affinity for M receptors but dissociates slowly from M1 and M3 subtype, resulting in prolonged (24 hour) bronchodilator effect.[23] Clinical trials in children show benefits in improving lung function and reducing exacerbations and an excellent safety profile.[24–26] Tiotropium is available in 2 doses via soft mist MDI (Respimat), 2.5 μg and 1.25 μg per actuation. Two puffs of the 1.25-μg dose administered once daily has been approved in the United States for children, although higher doses may be more effective. Peak effect on FEV_1 occurs within 1 to 3 hours after dosing. Whatever step-up therapy is used, attempts should be made at regular intervals (usually 3 months) to decrease the controller dose to the lowest level that adequately controls symptoms and exacerbations and maintains normal pulmonary function. Children in this category will benefit from referral to and possibly ongoing care from an asthma specialist.

Approximately 5% to 10% of children will have daily symptoms, frequent nocturnal awakenings, and a persistent obstructive defect measured by spirometry despite treatment with medium-dose ICS, plus another controller medication. Patients with such severe disease require high doses of ICS in combination with one or more other controller medications. If control is inadequate, oral corticosteroids are the next recommended treatment step. Following administration of a short course (<10 days) of daily dosing (1–2 mg/kg/d, maximum 40–60 mg prednisone) to stabilize symptoms, every-other-day treatment at the lowest-effective dose (0.5 mg/kg) will usually achieve control. Before instituting systemic steroid therapy, a thorough search for remediable exacerbating factors or comorbid conditions (discussed later) should be sought. As soon as symptoms are controlled, oral steroid dose should be tapered to lowest at which symptom control is maintained. A single morning dose is well tolerated and helps minimize systemic side effects, but children with severe or refractory symptoms may require twice-daily dosing. Chronic oral corticosteroid therapy requires careful monitoring for adverse effects, such as impaired linear growth, adrenal suppression, hypertension, cataract formation, hyperglycemia, and loss of bone mineral content.

A proportion of severe asthmatics may have relative steroid resistance, either acquired or due to a non-T2 endotype.[27] Such patients may have altered steroid metabolism or receptor dysfunction; pharmacokinetic and cellular studies may be helpful to diagnose the cause of the defect. Patients who are steroid resistant are candidates for alternative therapies, such as omalizumab, mepolizumab, or other immune modulators. Children with severe asthma should receive routine care from a specialist to assess symptom control, pulmonary function, medication adherence, comorbid conditions, and adverse effects caused by treatment. Severe asthma is discussed in more detail in Drs Angela Marko and Kristie R. Ross' article, "Severe Asthma in Childhood."

MANAGEMENT OF COMORBIDITIES

Asthma control may be difficult to assess in the setting of unrecognized or undertreated comorbidities. Escalating asthma treatments in these cases will not result in improvement in symptoms. Some comorbidities may be manifestations of related inflammatory processes outside the airway, whereas others are due to independent disease processes, exposures, or behaviors.

Obesity

Like asthma, its prevalence is more common among minorities; African American and Hispanic (particularly Puerto Rican) children are more commonly affected compared with their non-Hispanic white counterparts.[28] In defining asthma as an umbrella term, it appears that obesity-related asthma may be a distinct phenotype. Moreover, metabolic dysfunction in obesity, rather than body mass index, may be more closely related to asthma morbidity. Obesity has also been shown in several cross-sectional and prospective epidemiologic studies to be an independent risk factor for developing asthma.[28] Prospective cohort studies have shown a 2-fold increased risk of future asthma in obese children compared with normal weight children.[29] There are several proposed mechanisms that explain the association between asthma and obesity. The mechanical, or mass, impact on pulmonary function from excessive truncal adiposity can lead to a mechanical disadvantage to the diaphragm, with resultant decreased functional residual capacity (FRC), residual volume, and expiratory reserve volume. Lower FRC influences bronchial smooth muscle stretch, particularly at the end of a tidal breath, which subsequently leads to the perception of increased respiratory effort with inspiration. Obese children may have a higher absolute value for FEV_1 and forced vital capacity (FVC) and a lower FEV1/FVC ratio, in part related to airway dysynapsis; this finding is also associated with an increased risk of severe exacerbations.[30] Two studies have demonstrated the effect of weight loss on obesity-related asthma in children; weight loss is associated with improvement in clinical and quality-of-life parameters.[31,32] However, weight loss programs in children have only shown a modest effect and are rarely sustained. Obesity also has immunomodulatory effects as a low-grade inflammatory state. A subset of obese asthmatics has skewing CD4 cells toward Th1 cytokines.[33] This type of inflammation may then contribute to the obese asthmatic having less response to inhaled steroids and impaired disease control. More study is needed to elucidate mechanisms, pathways, and effective interventions for the obese-asthma phenotype.

Gastroesophageal Reflux

The association between asthma and gastroesophageal reflux disease (GERD) has long been debated, and the causal relationship between the 2 remains unclear.[34] Symptoms of gastroesophageal reflux (GER) and asthma tend to overlap, and both can result in nocturnal cough and sleep disturbances, as well as chest tightness, chest pressure, and chest pain. The exact mechanism explaining the association between GERD and asthma is unclear. Recurrent microaspiration into the upper airway may trigger a systemic inflammatory process and worsen asthma symptoms. In addition, there are pH-sensitive irritant receptors (present in both the esophagus and the trachea), that when stimulated lead to increased airway hyperresponsiveness and bronchospasm.[34] There have been relatively few clinical trials in the pediatric population to determine if the treatment of GERD results in improvement in asthma control.[35] One study demonstrated improved asthma control (less short-acting bronchodilator use) and severity (decrease in controller medication use).[36] However, this effect did not replicate in several other randomized, double-blind placebo-control studies. Another trial showed improvement in quality-of-life measures, but no other significant changes between study groups.[37] Another randomized clinical trial showed no improvement in asthma control or lung function in the treated group, but did show an increase in adverse events in the group treated with lansoprazole.[38] An evaluation for GER in patients with difficult to treat asthma is indicated but may be difficult to diagnose by history alone given overlap of symptoms. Data from a large double-blind clinical trial in children with symptomatic asthma demonstrated no improvement in any measure of asthma control with treatment with proton pump inhibitors (PPI) in patients who did not have symptoms of GER.[38] Given long-term risk of bone loss associated with PPI use,[39] medical reflux treatment in asthmatic children should be limited to those with clear diagnosis (symptoms and impedance probe testing) and symptoms not responsive to lifestyle/dietary changes.

Chronic Sinusitis

Sinusitis (or rhinosinusitis) describes a spectrum of infectious and inflammatory nasal symptoms, further classified as acute, subacute, or chronic based on duration of symptoms.[40] In the pediatric population, 20% to 30% of children with asthma have been found to have sinusitis on radiographic studies.[41,42] Acute sinusitis may be distinguished from typical upper respiratory tract infection by duration of symptoms beyond 1 to 20 days, with fever that persists or recurs beyond a few days, along with nasal congestion, facial, ear, or dental pain. Chronic sinusitis may have more persistent nasal symptoms without fever and be associated with worsening asthma symptoms. Chronic sinusitis may be caused by infection, allergic inflammation, and/or anatomic processes and associated with asthma severity.[43] Because of the impact of chronic sinusitis on asthma control, it is important to address underlying sinus disease, especially with nasal symptoms and disease that is poorly responsive to typical asthma therapies. Treatment of sinus disease may involve antibiotics, saline nasal rinses, and topical steroids.[44,45]

Allergen Rhinitis

In patients with asthma and allergic rhinitis (AR), upper airway inflammation cannot be viewed and treated in isolation, because the same inflammatory pathways may lead to both nasal allergy and asthma symptoms ("one-airway" model). AR and asthma often coexist. Data from the Tucson Children's Respiratory Study show that among atopic children with AR, the prevalence of asthma was 32%.[46] AR itself is an independent risk factor for the development of asthma.[47] There has been evidence of the early sensitization to multiple allergens associated with the greatest risk of asthma during childhood.[48,49] Although it does not appear that early treatment and interventions to decrease AR symptoms can stop development of asthma, treatment of AR can lead to some improvement in short-term asthma outcomes (improvement in control and decrease exacerbations).[50] Exposure to specific allergen triggers can not only worsen AR symptoms but also may lead to poor asthma control and increased use of asthma-related resources, especially in those sensitized to molds.[51] Management can be complicated by both exposure to unrecognized allergens and unrecognized exposure to known allergens. Allergy testing is an important part of identifying possible ongoing or unknown exposures. In addition, evaluation of the home environment may be indicated if allergy symptoms continue despite attempts to treat medically and eliminate exposures. Systemic antihistamines, topical nasal steroids, and antihistamines as well as LTRA have all been shown efficacious in treating AR. Allergen immunotherapy for those with refractory symptoms to certain inhalants (dust, grass, tree, ragweed) may also be helpful in controlling AR and possibly asthma.

Obstructive Sleep Apnea and Sleep-Disordered Breathing

Sleep-disordered breathing (SBD) is a broad term, which encompasses obstructive sleep apnea (OSA), central sleep apnea, hypoventilation disorders, as well as intermittent desaturations with snoring.[52,53] OSA occurs in 1% to 5% of children and is most commonly caused by upper airway obstruction due to tonsil and adenoid hypertrophy. Asthma and OSA commonly coexist, with a significant overlap in nocturnal symptoms, which may complicate the recognition and treatment of both disease processes. There does appear to be significant bidirectional interactions between the 2 conditions that lead to difficulty treating and controlling symptoms of both OSA and asthma.[52] SDB and asthma severity are also associated and appear to be independent of obesity.[53] The link between asthma and OSA is difficult to discuss in isolation, given the association between OSA and several other asthma-related comorbidities (GER, AR, and obesity). It is important to screen for symptoms of SDB, perform polysomnography if needed, and treat OSA (medical or surgical); however, the relationship between OSA treatment and improvement in asthma control needs further investigation.

Management of Comorbidities: Fungal Sensitization and Allergic Bronchopulmonary Aspergillosis

A rare but important asthma comorbidity is fungal sensitization. A wide variety of fungi have been implicated, with the most common being *Alternaria, Aspergillus, Penicillium,* and *Cladosporium.*[54] Fungal exposure and subsequent sensitization have an impact on asthma severity.[55] In particular, allergic bronchopulmonary aspergillosis (ABPA) can lead to loss of asthma control, worsening asthma severity, and development of bronchiectasis, particularly in those with atopic disease.[55] ABPA diagnosis requires recognition of clinical and immunologic features. ABPA usually occurs in the setting of worsening asthma, deterioration of lung function, *Aspergillus* skin test reactivity, serum IgE greater than 1000 ng/mL, increased *Aspergillus* species-specific IgE and IgG antibodies, and an abnormal chest radiograph.[54] Sensitization to *Aspergillus* without all other criteria for diagnosis of ABPA is common, especially in a child with atopic disease. Treatment of ABPA is typically an extended course of oral steroids, with or without systemic antifungal therapy; omalizumab has also been reported as a successful adjunct treatment.[56] Treatment of fungal sensitization asthma with anti-fungal agents remains controversial.[54]

Vocal Cord Dysfunction

Vocal cord dysfunction (VCD) or paradoxic vocal cord motion is defined as the involuntary adduction of the vocal cords during inspiration.[57] The prevalence of VCD in the pediatric population is difficult to determine, given that it is often misdiagnosed as poorly controlled asthma or EIB. VCD appears most commonly in the adolescent girl.[58] However, it can occur in the younger school-aged child and can lead to overtreatment of asthma symptoms if the diagnosis is missed. Symptoms include tightness in the throat ("throat closing") or upper chest, stridor (which is often mistaken for wheezing), and extreme shortness of breath. Exercise is a common trigger, along with AR, GER, and anxiety. Diagnosis is made based on history, presence of blunting of expiratory limb of flow volume loop, stridor during exercise challenge testing, or direct observation via laryngoscopy. Treatment includes speech therapy and addressing triggers.

PATIENT AND FAMILY EDUCATION

Adherence to medication is important to overall treatment and control of asthma. Without proper understanding of disease process and medications, it is difficult for families to adhere to therapy. Understanding parent and patient health care beliefs and promoting shared decision making are critical to improving adherence. Current asthma guidelines recommend use of a patient-specific asthma action plan in order to promote self-management.[6] Asthma action plans demonstrate some effect on improvement in adherence and asthma control, but other studies have not shown benefit compared with verbal instructions.[59–61] Addressing adherence and proper medication use must be an on-going conversation between the provider, patient, and family.

FUTURE CONSIDERATIONS/SUMMARY

Asthma is a complex heterogeneous disease that requires careful diagnosis to understand phenotypic differences that exist in school-aged children with asthma. Asthma management in school-aged children centers on pharmacologic treatment, addressing underlying comorbidities, and education of the patient and caregivers. Phenotypic differences and underlying comorbid conditions will impact pharmacologic treatment choices. Regular assessment of asthma control must be performed in order to appropriately manage the disorder.

REFERENCES

1. Akinbami L, Simon A, Rossen L. Changing trends in asthma prevalence among children. Pediatrics 2016;137(1):1–7.

2. Konradsen J, Skantz E, Nordlund B. Predicting asthma morbidity in children using proposed markers of Th2-type inflammation. Pediatr Allergy Immunol 2015; 26(8):772–9.

3. Just J, Saint Pierre P, Amat F. What lessons can be learned about asthma phenotypes in children from cohort studies? Pediatr Allergy Immunol 2015;26(4):300–5.
4. Randolph C. Pediatric exercise-induced bronchoconstriction: contemporary developments in epidemiology, pathogenesis, presentation, diagnosis, and therapy. Curr Allergy Asthma Rep 2013;13:662–71.
5. Global Initiative for Asthma. Global strategy for asthma management and prevention 2018. Available at: ginasthma.org. Accessed October 18, 2018.
6. Guidelines for the diagnosis and management of asthma. Available at: https://www.nhlbi.nih.gov/health-topics/guidelines-for-diagnosis-management-of-asthma. Accessed October 10, 2018.
7. Voorend-van Bergen S, Vaessen-Verberne A. Asthma control questionnaires in the management of asthma in children: a review. Pediatr Pulmonol 2015;50(2):202–8.
8. Nguyen J, Holbrook J, Wei C. Validation and psychometric properties of the asthma control questionnaire among children. J Allergy Clin Immunol 2014; 133(1):91–7.
9. Price D, Martin R, Barnes N, et al. Prescribing practices and asthma control with hydrofluoroalkane-beclomethasone and fluticasone: a real-world observational study. J Allergy Clin Immunol 2010;126:511–8.
10. Dinakar C, Oppenheimer J, Portnoy J, et al. Management of acute loss of asthma control in the yellow zone: a practice parameter. Ann Allergy Asthma Immunol 2014;113:143–59.
11. Martinez FD, Chinchilli V, Morgan W, et al. Use of beclomethasone dipropionate as rescue treatment for children with mild persistent asthma (TREXA): a randomized,double-blind, placebo-controlled trial. Lancet 2011;377:650–7.
12. Piacentini G, Peroni D, Bodini A, et al. Azithromycin reduces bronchial hyperresponsiveness and neutrophilic airway inflammation in asthmatic children: a preliminary report. Allergy Asthma Proc 2007;28:194–8.
13. Bacharier L, Guilbert T, Mauger D, et al. Early administration of azithromycin and prevention of severe lower respiratory tract illnesses in preschool children with a history of such illnesses: a randomized clinical trial. JAMA 2015;314:2034–44.
14. Lemanske R, Mauger D, Sorkness C, et al. Step-up therapy for children with uncontrolled asthma receiving inhaled corticosteroids. N Engl J Med 2010;362: 975–85.
15. Chauhan B, Ducharme F. Addition to inhaled corticosteroids of long-acting beta2-agonists versus anti-leukotrienes for chronic asthma. Cochrane Database Syst Rev 2014;(1):CD003137.
16. Vaessen-Verberne AA, Van den Berg NJ, Van Nierop JC, et al. Combination therapy salmeterol/fluticasone versus doubling dose of fluticasone in children with asthma. Am J Respir Crit Care Med 2010;182:1221–7.
17. Stempel D, Szefler S, Pedersen S, et al. Safety of adding salmeterol to fluticasone propionate in children with asthma. N Engl J Med 2016;375(9):840–9.
18. Sobieraj DM, Baker WL, Weeda ER, et al. Intermittent inhaled corticosteroids and long-acting muscarinic antagonists for asthma [Internet]. Review No. 194. (Prepared by the University of Connecticut Evidence-based Practice Center under Contract No. 290-2015-00012-I.) AHRQ Publication No. 17(18)-EHC027-EF. Rockville (MD): Agency for Healthcare Research and Quality; 2018.
19. O'Byrne PM, Bisgaard H, Godard PP, et al. Budesonide/formoterol combination therapy as both maintenance and reliever medication in asthma. Am J Respir Crit Care Med 2005;171(2):129–36.
20. Bisgaard H, Le Roux P, Bjåmer D, et al. Budesonide/formoterol maintenance plus reliever therapy: a new strategy in pediatric asthma. Chest 2006;130:1733–43.

21. Jackson D, Bacharier L, Mauger D, et al. Quintupling inhaled glucocorticoids to prevent childhood asthma exacerbations. N Engl J Med 2018;378(10):891–901.
22. Simons FE, Villa J, Lee B, et al. Montelukast added to budesonide in children with persistent asthma. A randomized double-blind, crossover study. J Pediatr 2001; 138:694–8.
23. Barnes P. Biochemical basis of asthma therapy. J Biol Chem 2011;286:899–905.
24. Vogelberg C, Moroni-Zentgraf P, Leoaviciute-Klimantaviciene M, et al. A randomized dose-ranging study of tiotropium Respimat in children with symptomatic asthma depside inhaled corticosteroids. Respir Res 2015.
25. Szefler S, Murphy K, Harper T, et al. A phase III randomized controlled trial of tiotropium add-on therapy in children with severe symptomatic asthma. J Allergy Clin Immunol 2017;140(5):1277–87.
26. Hamelmann E, Szefler S. Efficacy and safety of tiotropium in children and adolescents. Drugs 2018;78(3):327–38.
27. Chambers E, Nanzer A, Pfeffer P, et al. Distinct endotypes of steroid-resistant asthma characterized by IL-17A(high) and IFN-γ(high) immunophenotypes: Potential benefits of calcitriol. J Allergy Clin Immunol 2015;136:628–37.
28. Ford E. The epidemiology of obesity and asthma. J Allergy Clin Immunol 2005; 115(5):897–909.
29. Chen Y, Dong G, Lin K, et al. Gender difference of childhood overweight and obesity in predicting the risk of incident asthma: a systematic review and meta-analysis. Obes Rev 2013;14(3):222–31.
30. Forno E, Weiner D, Mullen J, et al. Obesity and airway dysanapsis in children with and without asthma. Am J Respir Crit Care Med 2017;195(3):314–23.
31. Luna-Pech J, Torres-Mendoza B, Garcia-Cobas C, et al. Normocaloric diet improves asthma-related quality of life in obese pubertal adolescents. Int Arch Allergy Immunol 2014;163:252–8.
32. Van Leeuwen J, Hoogstrate M, Duiverman E, et al. Effects of dietary induced weight loss on exercise-induced bronchoconstriction in overweight and obese children. Pediatr Pulmonol 2014;49:1155–61.
33. Vijayakanthi N, Greally JM, Rastogi D. Pediatric obesity-related Athma: the role of metabolic dysregulation. Pediatrics 2016;137(5):1–16.
34. Blake K, Teague WG. Gastroesophageal reflux disease and childhood asthma. Curr Opin Pulm Med 2013;19(1):24–9.
35. Miceli Sopa S, Radzik D, Calvani M. Does treatment with proton pump inhibitors for gastroesphogeal reflux disease (GERD) improve asthma symptoms in children with asthma and GERD? A systematic review. J Investig Allergol Clin Immunol 2009;19(1):1–5.
36. Khoshoo V, Le T, Haydel RM, et al. Role of gastroesophageal relfux in older children with asthma. Chest 2003;123(4):1008–13.
37. Stordal K, Johannesdottir G, Bentsen B. Acid suppression does not change respiratory symptoms in children with asthma and gastroesophageal reflux disease. Arch Dis Child 2005;90:956–60.
38. Holdbrook J, Wise R, Gold B. Lansoprazole for children with poorly controlled asthma: a randomized clinical trial. JAMA 2012;307:373–81.
39. Ali T, Roberts DN, Tierney WM. Long-term safety concerns with proton pump inhibitors. Am J Med 2009;122(10):896–903.
40. Lai L, Hopp R, Lusk R. Pediatric chronic sinusitis and asthma: a review. J Asthma 2006;43:719–25.
41. Rachelefsky G, Goldberg M, Katz R, et al. Sinus disease in children with respiratory allergy. J Allergy Clin Immunol 1978;61:310–4.

42. Zimmerman B, Stringer D, Feanny S, et al. Prevalence of abnormalities found by sinus x-rays in childhood asthma: lack of relation to severity of asthma. J Allergy Clin Immunol 1987;80:268–83.
43. Lin D, Chandra R, Tan B, et al. Association between severity of asthma and degree of chronic rhinosinusitis. Am J Rhinol Allergy 2011;25(4):205–8.
44. Chow A, Benninger M, Brook I, et al. IDSA clinical practice guideline for acute bacterial rhinosinusitis in children and adults. Clin Infect Dis 2012;54(8):e72–112.
45. Chandran S, Higgins T. Pediatric rhinosinusitis: definintions, diagnosis, and management- an overview. Am J Rhinol Allergy 2013;1(3):16–9.
46. Wright A, Holberg C, Martinez F, et al. Epidemiology of physician-diagnosed allergic rhinitis in childhood. Pediatrics 1994;94(6):895–901.
47. Togias A. Rhinitis and asthma: evidence for respiratory system integration. J Allergy Clin Immunol 2003;111(6):1171–83.
48. Havstad S, Johnson CC, Kim H, et al. Atopic phenotypes identified with latent class analyses at age 2 years. J Allergy Clin Immunol 2014;134(3):722–7.
49. Rubner FJ, Jackson DJ, Evans MD, et al. Early life rhinovirus wheezing, allergic sensitization, and asthma risk at adolescence. J Allergy Clin Immunol 2017; 139(2):501–7.
50. Tsilochristou O, Douladiris N, Makris M, et al. Pediatric allergic rhinitis and asthma: can the march be halted? Paediatr Drugs 2013;15(6):431–40.
51. Denning DW, O'Driscoll BR, Hogaboam CM, et al. The link between fungi and severe asthma: as summary of the evidence. Eur Respir J 2006;27(3):615–26.
52. Min YZ, Subbarao P, Narang I. The bidirectional relationship between asthma and obstructive sleep apnea: which came first? J Pediatr 2016;176:10–6.
53. Ross K, Storfer-Isser A, Hart M, et al. Sleep-disordered breathing is associated with asthma severity in children. J Pediatr 2012;160(5):736–42.
54. Knutsen A, Bush R, Demain J, et al. Fungi and allergic lower respiratory tract disease. J Allergy Clin Immunol 2012;129(2):280–93.
55. Ghosh S, Hoselton S, Schuh J. Allergic inflammation in *Aspergillus fumigatus*-induced fungal asthma. Curr Allergy Asthma Rep 2015;15:1–11.
56. Moss R. The use of biological agents for the treatment of fungal asthma and allergic bronchopulmonary aspergillosis. Ann N Y Acad Sci 2012;1272:49–57.
57. Fretzayas A, Moustaki M, Loukou I, et al. Differentiating vocal cord dysfunction from asthma. J Asthma Allergy 2017;10:277–83.
58. Maturo S, Hill C, Buntin G. Pediatric paradoxical vocal-fold motion: presentation and natural history. Pediatrics 2011;128(6):e1443–9.
59. Agrawal S, Singh M, Mathew J, et al. Efficacy of an individualized written home-management plan in the control of moderate persistent asthma: a randomized, controlled trial. Acta Paediatr 2005;94:1742–6.
60. Ducharme F, Zemek R, Chalut D, et al. Written action plan in pediatric emergency room improves asthma prescribing, adherence, and control. Am J Respir Crit Care Med 2011;183:195–203.
61. Sheares B, Mellins R, Dimango E, et al. Do patients of subspecialist physicians benefit from written asthma action plans? Am J Respir Crit Care Med 2015; 191(12):1374–83.

Recent Diagnosis Techniques in Pediatric Asthma

Impulse Oscillometry in Preschool Asthma and Use of Exhaled Nitric Oxide

Karen M. McDowell, MD

KEYWORDS

- Preschool asthma • Pulmonary function testing • Impulse oscillometry • Impedance
- Resistance • Reactance • Coherence • Tidal breathing

KEY POINTS

- Objective measures of lung function are important in the diagnosis and management of asthma, yet most preschoolers cannot perform spirometry.
- Impulse oscillometry, which is performed during tidal breathing, is a method by which lung function measures can be obtained in preschool children.
- Impulse oscillometry can be useful in determining baseline lung function, demonstrating response to bronchodilator or bronchoprovocation, and predicting asthma exacerbations and loss of disease control.
- Fractional exhaled nitric oxide (FeNO) levels reflect eosinophilic inflammation and predict responsiveness to corticosteroids.
- Although FeNO has been used to discriminate among wheezing phenotypes, the role of FeNO in preschool wheezing remains unclear.

INTRODUCTION

Objective assessment of lung function is important in the diagnosis of asthma and assessment of disease control.[1] Spirometry is the pulmonary function test most widely used to evaluate for airway obstruction in children and is recommended as part of asthma evaluation and management by both US[1] and European guidelines.[2] Spirometry requires a child to be able to follow directions and perform maximal respiratory maneuvers, such as full inspiration to total lung capacity and forced exhalation to residual volume, ideally over 6 seconds. In addition, the child must be able to provide

Disclosure: Dr K.M. McDowell has no financial or commercial conflicts of interest regarding the material contained within this article.

Division of Pulmonary Medicine, Cincinnati Children's Hospital Medical Center, Department of Pediatrics, University of Cincinnati College of Medicine, 3333 Burnet Avenue, MLC 7041, Cincinnati, OH 45229, USA

E-mail address: karen.mcdowell@cchmc.org

Immunol Allergy Clin N Am 39 (2019) 205–219
https://doi.org/10.1016/j.iac.2018.12.002
0889-8561/19/© 2018 Elsevier Inc. All rights reserved.

reproducible efforts. Children less than 5 years of age are rarely able to perform such a skilled, effort-dependent test. Thus, preschool asthma is most often diagnosed and managed based on clinical findings. Although not as readily available as spirometry, impulse oscillometry (IOS) is a lung function test that can be performed by younger children and those unable to perform spirometry to provide important objective information in those diagnosed with or suspected to have asthma.

IMPULSE OSCILLOMETRY

Because IOS requires minimal cooperation and measurements are made during tidal breathing, it is an ideal method for assessing lung function in preschool children. It has been performed reliably and consistently even by children unable to perform spirometry.[3,4] However, a recent large multicenter study of inner-city children at risk for asthma found that of 485 children who attempted lung function testing, a higher percentage was able to perform acceptable spirometry than IOS at ages 3, 4, and 5 years.[5] It is worth noting, though, that the study used forced expiratory volume in 0.5 second ($FEV_{0.5}$) rather than the more commonly used forced expiratory volume in 1 second (FEV_1) in determining acceptable and repeatable spirometry. Nevertheless, these investigators and others have shown IOS to be more sensitive than spirometry in detecting small-airway obstruction and distinguishing children with asthma from those who did not.[6–9] IOS has also shown utility in not only identifying inadequate asthma control[10] but also predicting future loss of control and asthma exacerbations.[11,12] An additional advantage of IOS is that it can measure airway resistance, which cannot be obtained through spirometry and typically requires body plethysmography.

IOS is a form of the forced oscillation technique described in 1956 by Dubois and colleagues.[13] Forced oscillation measures airway mechanics by superimposing pressure waves on the subject's tidal breathing. IOS uses sound waves to transmit pressure into the airways and thereby determine pressure and flow over a range of frequencies. Once pressure and flow have been determined, other characteristics of the airway, such as resistance, can be calculated. Sound waves of lower frequencies (<15 Hz) travel deeper into the airways, allowing measurement of small-airway parameters. Higher-frequency sound waves are of higher amplitude and move over a shorter distance. Thus, measurements derived from sound waves with a frequency of greater than 20 Hz reflect large airway characteristics. By obtaining measurements over both high and low frequencies, IOS can reflect function of both proximal and distal airways.

Commercially available IOS systems contain a loudspeaker that generates sound waves over a range of frequencies, usually 2 to 35 Hz. The loudspeaker is attached to a mouthpiece, through which the oscillations of the sound and the concomitant pressure fluctuations are transmitted into the oropharynx, through the glottis, and into the lower airways. A pneumotachograph and transducer are connected to the tubing between the loudspeaker and the mouthpiece, allowing measurement of pressure and flow during inspiration and expiration. The generated sound waves are superimposed on the normal tidal breathing of the child, and a signal filter separates the externally produced oscillations from those of the child's breathing pattern. Computer analysis of amplitude and phase differences of pressure and flow during inspiration and expiration calculates respiratory impedance. Impedance of the respiratory system comprises all the forces that inhibit airflow.

CONCEPTS IN IMPULSE OSCILLOMETRY

Several concepts, including *impedance*, are important in understanding IOS. Total respiratory system impedance, represented as *Zrs*, is composed of *resistance (Rrs)* and *reactance (Xrs)*. Resistance can be conceptualized as the energy a sound wave requires to travel through the airways and inflate the lung. The resistance of the entire respiratory system (Rrs) includes that found in the extrathoracic airways, intrathoracic airways, lung parenchyma, and the chest wall. The resistance at low frequencies, such as 5 Hz (R5), is that of both the central and the distal airways, whereas resistance at higher frequencies such as 20 Hz (R20) represents that of the large airways. Resistance of the peripheral airways can be determined by subtracting resistance of the large airways from that of the respiratory system, or R5 − R20. This value is commonly referred to as the *R5-R20*. Peripheral airway obstruction results in more resistance in the lower-frequency sound waves (R5), which travel deeper into the lungs than the higher-frequency waves (R20) representing the large airways. Thus, R5 will be disproportionately elevated relative to R20 in peripheral airway obstruction, and consequently, a higher value for R5-R20 is obtained under such circumstances. This disproportionate effect on low-frequency resistance compared with high-frequency resistance in small-airway obstruction is called *frequency dependence of resistance*, which is an alternate term for R5-R20. In small-airway obstruction, the value of both R5 (resistance at low frequencies representing large and small airways) and R5-R20 (resistance of more peripheral airways) will be elevated.

Reactance of the respiratory system, represented as Xrs, is composed of the inert and elastic properties of the respiratory system. The elastic properties of the pulmonary system are manifested as the elastic recoil of the airways and lung parenchyma in response to distension. Reactance is the energy generated by the elastic recoil of the lung parenchyma and the airways added to the inertance of the system. Inertance is the force opposing movement of the sound wave through the respiratory system. Reactance can also be thought of as the "stored energy" of the respiratory system or rebound energy that is generated in response to the sound wave moving through the lungs. In contrast, resistance is the pressure opposing the forward movement of the sound wave and is a force occurring in front of and in phase with the sound wave. Reactance occurs in response to the sound wave and therefore is the energy echoed back to the system after, and out of phase with, the sound wave. The sum of the forces ahead of the sound wave (resistance) and those generated behind the sound wave in response to the pressure of the wave (reactance) equal the impedance of the entire respiratory system. In other words, Rrs + Xrs = Zrs. Inertance is the force opposing movement of the sound wave through the respiratory system. At low frequencies where sound waves have reached the more distal airways, elastic recoil (reactance) will be high compared with inertance. At higher frequencies, where sound waves travel only as far as the larger, more proximal, airways, elastic recoil (reactance) will be low compared with the inertive properties of the airways. It is not surprising then that reactance at low frequencies has been shown to correlate with peripheral airway obstruction.[14] When reactance is zero (X = 0), the elastic recoil of the airways and lungs is equal and opposite to the inertance of the system, and all of the impedance in the system is created by the forward movement of the sound wave. At this frequency, known as *resonant frequency* or *Fres*, low-frequency and high-frequency reactance can be discriminated. At frequencies above Fres, inertance is greater than elastic recoil as is seen in the large airways. Frequencies below Fres will be those at which elastic recoil is greater than inertance, a property of the small airways. Therefore, Fres is the dividing point between large and small airways based on the mechanical properties of the airways. It is important to realize that the distinction between large and small airways based on Fres is determined by the airway mechanics rather than the size or generation of the airway.[14] The value of Fres is higher in children than in adults and decreases with age.[15] Fres is also increased in airway obstruction.[16,17]

During IOS testing, curves for the resistance and reactance at all frequencies between 5 and 20 Hz are generated. Both curves are then plotted against frequency
and displayed on a single graph called a Goldman graph[4] (**Fig. 1**). The area under
the reactance curve between the values at 5 Hz (X5) and at Fres is called the *area of
reactance (AX)*. Both AX and X5 provide information about distal airway obstruction
because reactance (elastic recoil) is greatest in the small airways, where low-
frequency sound waves can reach. Obstruction of the small airways results in lower
(more negative) values for X5 (reduced reactance or elastic recoil). Similarly, the Fres
is higher in airway obstruction because the point in the airways where reactance (elastic
recoil) is zero is more proximal, and the more proximal, larger airways are represented
by values obtained at higher frequencies. Lower X5 and/or higher Fres will increase the
area under the reactance curve, and therefore, the value of AX. It follows then that AX is
elevated in proportion to small-airway obstruction.[18,19] AX has been reported to be the
most sensitive measure in discriminating between asthmatics and healthy controls.[6,9]

A final concept is that of *coherence*. Coherence is based on the ratio of the pressure
of the sound wave entering the lung and the pressure of its reflection back from the
respiratory system. Coherence is measured in units of cm H_2O between 0 and 1.

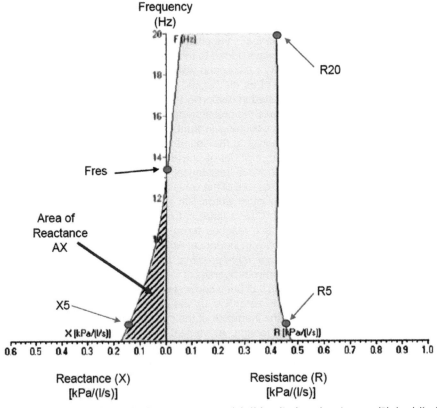

Fig. 1. A Goldman graph displaying reactance (X) (*blue line*) and resistance (R) (*red line*)
plotted as a function of frequency. Fres is the frequency where X = 0. X5 and R5 are reactance
at 5 Hz and resistance at 5 Hz, respectively. The AX is the shaded triangle represented by the
area under the reactance curve between Fres and 0 Hz. R5, Fres, and AX will be increased in
peripheral airway obstruction. X5 will be more negative in peripheral airway obstruction.

Perfect coherence, where the pressure of the entering sound wave is equal to the pressure of the echoing sound wave, is valued at 1 cm H_2O. Hence, coherence can be used as a measure of the quality or validity of the IOS measurements with coherence closer to 1 representing better validity. In general, a coherence of ≥ 0.8 is acceptable.

OBTAINING IMPULSE OSCILLOMETRY MEASUREMENTS

IOS may be performed with the child seated in a chair or seated on the parent's lap. Legs must be uncrossed to prevent contraction of the abdominal muscles, which can result in lower-end expiratory lung volumes. Nose clips are used to prevent leakage of pressure through the nose. With the head in neutral position, the child places the mouthpiece into his or her mouth and makes a seal with the lips. The cheeks are supported by an adult to prevent shifting of impulses to the upper airway and to limit the compliance of the cheeks.[20,21] Sound waves are generated by the loudspeaker while the child performs tidal breathing for 20 to 30 seconds. Rrs and Xrs are measured and displayed in real time for inspection by the operator. Rrs and Xrs for all frequencies between 5 and 20 Hz are derived and stored for each trial. A minimum of 3 acceptable trials with less than 10% variation among trials are performed. All equipment calibration and testing should be done in accordance with American Thoracic Society (ATS)/European Respiratory Society standards.[20] The performance of the test takes only a few minutes; however, in young children, additional time should be allowed for acclimation to the equipment and testing environment before the IOS procedure is performed.

REFERENCE VALUES FOR IMPULSE OSCILLOMETRY

Reference values in spirometry are affected predominantly by height, but also by age, gender, race, and ethnicity, and predicted normal values are accessible for diverse racial and ethnic groups. In contrast, predicted values in IOS are also based principally on height but are derived from an ethnically homogeneous sample, which is largely white. The equations are based almost exclusively on data obtained from white children of European descent.[22–25] However, a literature review by Galant and colleagues[26] and subsequent comparison of values obtained from diverse populations and commercially available regression equations revealed that normative values for R5 and X5 in healthy children and adults are comparable despite differences in geographic and ethnic origin, and these values correlate with the values obtained from regression equations programmed into commercially available software. Thus, predicted values programmed into commercially available software should be considered reasonable reference values for R5 and X5. Unfortunately, because of a paucity of data, there is still a need to establish reference values for other important IOS parameters, such as AX.

INTERPRETATION OF IMPULSE OSCILLOMETRY

The most commonly used parameters in interpretation of IOS are R5, R20, X5, Fres, and AX. Values for R5 and R20 that are greater than 150% of predicted should be considered abnormal and are consistent with increased airway resistance. An R5-R20 value is considered elevated, and consistent with peripheral airway obstruction, if it is greater than 30% in children and greater than 20% in adults. The within-individual variability of airway resistance when measured by IOS is approximately 16% for children and 10% for adults, which is comparable to the 5% to 15% individual variability in airway resistance obtained by body plethysmography.[22]

Decreasing values for X5 indicate a loss of elastic recoil to the system at 5 Hz as would be present in peripheral airway obstruction. X5 is abnormal if the value is greater than 150% of predicted. The Fres (where reactance is zero), is abnormal if it is greater than 25 Hz in children or greater than 20 Hz in adults. A higher value for Fres indicates increased resistance. Fres naturally decreases with age. There are no accepted reference values for AX.

IOS measurements are considered accurate when coherence at 5 Hz is greater than 0.8 and coherence at 20 Hz is between 0.9 and 1.[27,28] Causes of decreased coherence include swallowing, glottis closure, coughing, mouthpiece obstruction by the tongue, or irregular respiratory pattern. The parameters measured in IOS, their definitions, and normal values are summarized in **Table 1**.

IMPULSE OSCILLOMETRY AND ASTHMA

One of the most useful areas of application for IOS is pediatric asthma. IOS can provide objective measures of lung function even in children who cannot perform spirometry,

Table 1
Description, abbreviations, and normal values for common impulse oscillometry parameters

IOS Parameter	Symbol	Description	Reference Values
Respiratory impedance	Zrs	Impedance = resistance + reactance	
Respiratory resistance	Rrs	Airway + tissue + chest wall resistance	
	R5	Resistance at frequency of 5 Hz = resistance of proximal and distal airways	R5 normal if ≤150% predicted
	R20	Resistance at frequency of 20 Hz = resistance of proximal airways	R20 normal if ≤150% predicted
	R5-R20	Value at R5 – value at R20 = resistance of small airways	None established but increase suggestive of elevated small-airway resistance
Respiratory reactance	Xrs	Elastic + inertive properties of airways + lung tissue	
	X5	Reactance at frequency of 5 Hz Increased value suggests small-airway obstruction	Abnormal if X5 >150% predicted
Resonant frequency	Fres	Frequency at which elastic forces = inertive forces; X = 0 Increased value suggests peripheral airway obstruction	Adults: Normal <12 Hz Abnormal >20 Hz Children: Normal <20–25 Hz Abnormal >25 Hz
Reactance area	AX	Area under the reactance curve bounded by Fres and X5 Increased value suggests peripheral airway obstruction	None established but increase suggestive of peripheral airway obstruction
Coherence	Co Co 5 Co 20	Indicator of quality control Assessment of reproducibility Coherence at 5 Hz Coherence at 20 Hz	Test acceptable if: Co 5 Hz 0.7–0.9 Co 20 Hz 0.9–1.0

allowing earlier detection of airway obstruction and response to treatment. IOS has been studied extensively in asthma, including during acute exacerbations. Children with asthma have elevated resistance, specifically R5, as well as decreased Xrs at baseline compared with children without asthma,[8,29] and R20 and Fres have also been shown to be increased in asthmatics compared with healthy controls[9,30,31] (**Figs. 2 and 3**). Response to bronchodilator is the hallmark of bronchial hyperreactivity and a diagnostic criterion for asthma (see **Figs. 2** and **3**). Following administration of a bronchodilator, children with asthma demonstrate a decrease in resistance, both R5 and R5-R20, and in Xrs and AX.[7,8] However, the degree of response to bronchodilator reported has varied widely, anywhere from 8.6%[6] to more than 40%.[15] A review of pediatric studies revealed that when change greater than the upper limit of the 95% confidence interval for R5 is used, the mean bronchodilator response (BDR) in healthy children was 39%.[26] Thus, a decrease in R5 or X5 greater than or equal to 40% following administration of a bronchodilator should be considered a positive response in pediatric asthma. Even lower BDR cutoff values have been shown to distinguish between children with asthma and healthy controls. A BDR decrease of 20% in R5 or R10 differentiated asthmatic preschoolers from those without asthma.[28,32] Similarly, decreases of 8.6% at R10 and 29.1% in AX were found to identify asthma in school-aged children.[7] These same studies demonstrated changes in IOS parameters even without concomitant change in spirometry, indicating that IOS may be more sensitive than spirometry in distinguishing asthma from healthy controls. This increased sensitivity is most likely because IOS reflects changes in the caliber of the small airways where changes of asthma occur earlier, before the abnormalities in the larger airways characterized by spirometry.[11]

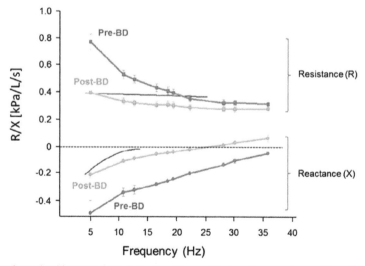

Fig. 2. Prebronchodilator and postbronchodilator IOS showing resistance (R) and reactance (X) plotted against frequency (Hz). At 5 Hz, there was 48% improvement in resistance and 58% improvement in reactance after 2 puffs (400 mg) of albuterol. There was a 23% decrease in resistance at 20 Hz. The R5-R20, which reflects peripheral airway resistance, improved from 75% to 58% after bronchodilator (BD). Measurements were made using Tremoflo airway oscillometry. (*Courtesy of* Thorasys, Montreal, Quebec, Canada; and *From* Galant SP, Komarow HD, Hye-Won S, et al. The case for impulse oscillometry in the management of asthma in children and adults. Ann Allergy Asthma Immunol 2017;118(6):667; with permission.)

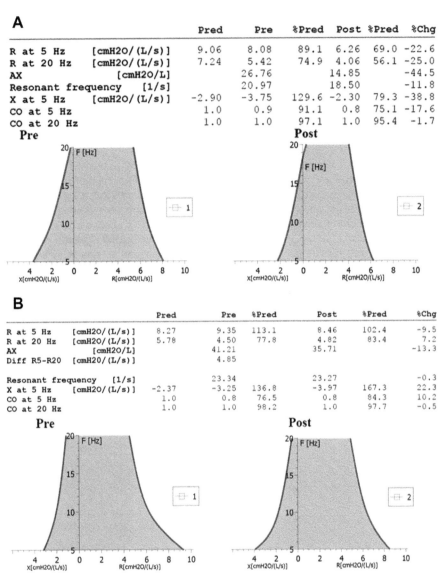

A

		Pred	Pre	%Pred	Post	%Pred	%Chg
R at 5 Hz	[cmH2O/(L/s)]	9.06	8.08	89.1	6.26	69.0	-22.6
R at 20 Hz	[cmH2O/(L/s)]	7.24	5.42	74.9	4.06	56.1	-25.0
AX	[cmH2O/L]		26.76		14.85		-44.5
Resonant frequency	[1/s]		20.97		18.50		-11.8
X at 5 Hz	[cmH2O/(L/s)]	-2.90	-3.75	129.6	-2.30	79.3	-38.8
CO at 5 Hz		1.0	0.9	91.1	0.8	75.1	-17.6
CO at 20 Hz		1.0	1.0	97.1	1.0	95.4	-1.7

Pre   Post

B

		Pred	Pre	%Pred	Post	%Pred	%Chg
R at 5 Hz	[cmH2O/(L/s)]	8.27	9.35	113.1	8.46	102.4	-9.5
R at 20 Hz	[cmH2O/(L/s)]	5.78	4.50	77.8	4.82	83.4	7.2
AX	[cmH2O/L]		41.21		35.71		-13.3
Diff R5-R20	[cmH2O/(L/s)]		4.85				
Resonant frequency	[1/s]		23.34		23.27		-0.3
X at 5 Hz	[cmH2O/(L/s)]	-2.37	-3.25	136.8	-3.97	167.3	22.3
CO at 5 Hz		1.0	0.8	76.5	0.8	84.3	10.2
CO at 20 Hz		1.0	1.0	98.2	1.0	97.7	-0.5

Pre   Post

Fig. 3. (A) IOS from a 6-year-old girl with chronic cough and normal spirometry without BDR. IOS reveals normal resistance (R) at 5 Hz and 20 Hz but decreased reactance at 5 Hz and increased AX. These results indicate peripheral airway obstruction. Following administration of bronchodilator, she had a 44.5% decrease in AX and 39% decrease in X5 signifying a positive response to bronchodilator. (B) IOS results from a 9-year-old boy with a history of corrected double aortic arch, tracheomalacia, and suspected asthma. Spirometry was persistently abnormal with flow volume loop suggestive of intrathoracic obstruction. IOS shows normal resistance at 5 Hz and 20 Hz. Reactance at 5 Hz is mildly decreased. There was no significant change in any parameter after bronchodilator. (*From* Bickel S, Popler J, Lesnick B, et al. Impulse oscillometry: interpretation and practical applications. Chest 2014;146(3):845; with permission.)

Investigators have also examined change in IOS parameters after bronchoprovocation tests. Schulze and colleagues[33] evaluated IOS and spirometry during methacholine challenge in 48 children with recurrent wheezing. In the 28 children who had significant changes in both FEV_1 and R5 during the challenge, a lower provocation dose was needed to attain a decrease in R5 than to achieve a 20% decrease in FEV_1,[34] implying that IOS may be more sensitive than spirometry in detecting response to methacholine. The investigators also noted that a 45% increase in R5 and/or a decrease in X5 of 0.69 kPa s L^{-1} predicted a 20% decrease in FEV_1 with adequate sensitivity and specificity. Peripheral airway resistance measurements after methacholine, especially R5-R20, have also been shown to significantly correlate with asthma severity.[34] Accordingly, IOS may be more helpful than spirometry in identifying children with more severe disease.

Shi and colleagues[10] studied lung function by spirometry and IOS in more than 100 healthy and asthmatic children. They demonstrated R5-R20 and AX to be useful and more sensitive than spirometry in identifying poorly controlled asthma. In a subsequent study of children with well-controlled asthma (based on clinical and spirometric measures), R5-R20 and AX predicted loss of disease control within 8 to 12 weeks better than spirometry, even when including measurements of forced expiratory flow between the 25th and 75th percentile of forced vital capacity (FVC).[12] A 1-year study of 4- to 7-year-old children with asthma revealed that R5 and R5-R20 were more predictive of asthma exacerbation than FEV_1, FEV_1/forced vital capacity, or methacholine challenge, and that IOS could identify with 80% accuracy which children would have exacerbations.[11] A recent report by Knihtilä and colleagues[35] determined that abnormalities in IOS measurements of R5 and R5-R20 at age 2 to 7 years were predictive of persistently abnormal FEV_1 after bronchodilator in adolescence. Thus, IOS may allow early detection of peripheral airway obstruction and provide opportunity for intervention to prevent additional decline in lung function.

FRACTIONAL EXHALED NITRIC OXIDE

Measurement of fractional exhaled nitric oxide (FeNO) is a noninvasive technique used to determine eosinophilic airway inflammation and has been studied as a tool to assist with the diagnosis and management of asthma. Nitric oxide (NO) is produced by respiratory epithelial cells, and production is increased in response to inflammatory cytokines in the airways.[36] In addition, NO results in dilatation of both blood vessels and airways in the human lung.[37] NO is present in exhaled breath, and measurements correlate with sputum eosinophil level.[38] Importantly, FeNO levels are elevated in children with asthma compared with those without asthma.[39,40] Because FeNO can be easily measured in children and reflects eosinophilic airway inflammation, it has significant potential to be useful in the diagnosis and management of asthma in children, especially those too young to perform spirometry. The ATS published an official Clinical Practice Guideline in 2011 addressing use of FeNO for diagnosis of eosinophilic airway inflammation.[41]

REFERENCE VALUES FOR FRACTIONAL EXHALED NITRIC OXIDE

An FeNO value greater than 50 parts per billion (ppb) is consistent with eosinophilic airway inflammation and an indication of responsiveness to corticosteroids; however, in children younger than 12 years old, the cutoff may be as low as 35 ppb. Values less than 20 ppb imply that little to no eosinophilic inflammation is present and are considered to be in the normal range.[41] In fact, a study of 150 children demonstrated that using a level of less than 20 ppb as normal had a sensitivity of 86%, specificity of 89%, positive predictive value of 92%, and negative predictive value of 80%.[40] Other investigators found increased risk of asthma and low false positive rates of asthma diagnosis for similar cutoff values.[42–44] Clinical information, such as recent use of inhaled or systemic steroids, is important in interpreting the significance of FeNO, especially intermediate FeNO levels (those between 20 and 35 ppb).

There is more variability in the mean levels reported among studies of FeNO in healthy infants and toddlers than in older children and adults. Meyts and colleagues[45] measured FeNO during tidal breathing in 89 healthy 4-year-old children and found the mean level of NO was 13 ± 0.4 ppb. A larger study of 121 normal children from 2 to 7 years of age yielded a mean tidal NO level of 3.0 (95% confidence interval 2.7–3.3) ppb.[46] More recently, a study of 53 healthy children ages 1 to 5 years without current asthma, history of asthma, viral wheezing, allergic rhinitis, eczema, other chronic airway disease, or active respiratory infection and who were not receiving any respiratory medications found a mean FeNO level of 7.1 ppb during tidal breathing (95% CI, 2.8–11.5 ppb).[47] Larger studies are needed to determine normative values for healthy infant and preschoolers.

There are numerous factors that influence FeNO values, including age, sex, height, atopy, smoking (active or passive exposure to tobacco smoke), consumption of nitrite-containing foods or caffeine,[48,49] and prematurity.[50,51] Thus, these factors must be taken into consideration when interpreting FeNO. Testing technique and analyzer type can also affect FeNO levels.[41] However, in children from 1 to 5 years of age, height, weight, age, and sex have been shown not to affect FeNO.[47] Prematurity has been shown to decrease FeNO levels.[50,51]

FRACTIONAL EXHALED NITRIC OXIDE AND DIAGNOSIS OF ASTHMA

Measurement of exhaled NO may be useful early in life to determine risk for developing asthma because eosinophilic airway inflammation precedes other criteria for the diagnosis of asthma.[52] However, FeNO has been shown to be elevated in conditions other than asthma and in both atopic and nonatopic children. For example, in children with recurrent wheezing, FeNO is significantly higher in those who have a positive Asthma Predictive Index (API) compared with those with a negative API (even though the median levels were low in both groups)[53,54] and children with no wheezing.[55] FeNO is higher for children with allergic asthma compared with nonallergic asthma[56] but also in those with allergic sensitization even without asthma.[56–58]

Despite the overlap in asthma and allergy in producing elevated FeNO, an association between high FeNO levels in childhood and subsequent asthma diagnosis has been reported by several investigators. The Prevention and Incidence of Asthma and Mite Allergy study, a large birth cohort study of 848 children from the Netherlands, demonstrated that elevated FeNO at age 4 is associated with increased physician-diagnosed asthma at age 7.[59] Similar results were found in a prospective study by Singer and colleagues.[60] Interestingly, FeNO levels are higher in children with bronchial hyperresponsiveness regardless of atopic status.[57,61]

FeNO has also been shown to distinguish among wheezing phenotypes in infants, preschoolers, and school-aged children. Gouvis-Echraghi and colleagues[62] reported that among children less than 3 years of age, those with uncontrolled, nonatopic moderate to severe asthma had the highest levels of exhaled NO. Children with viral-induced wheezing had the lowest levels of FeNO, and those with atopic wheezing had values intermediate to the other 2 wheezing phenotypes. Although FeNO represents eosinophilic inflammation that is typically responsive to steroids, in this population of 79 children, those whose asthma was uncontrolled despite use of ICS had the highest FeNO levels. Another investigation of FeNO levels in a large cohort of more than 970 children revealed the highest levels in subjects with late-onset wheezing.[63] The association between FeNO level and wheezing phenotype was present at age 4 but was even greater by 8 years of age. The same study reported that among atopic children, FeNO was higher in those with transient or occasional wheezing. It is clear that more investigation is necessary in order to understand the role of FeNO measurements in younger children given the complexity of preschool wheezing.

SUMMARY AND FUTURE CONSIDERATIONS

In summary, IOS is a method of obtaining objective measures of lung function in preschool children and others unable to perform spirometry. It is easily performed even by very young children because the test is performed during tidal breathing. IOS measures lung function in both the proximal and the peripheral airways and thereby is more sensitive to detecting airway obstruction and response to bronchodilator than spirometry. Airway resistance measurements that are not available through spirometry are a seminal feature of IOS. Furthermore, the resistance measurements obtained through IOS do not need to be corrected for lung volume, unlike resistance measurements made by plethysmography. IOS has demonstrated utility in distinguishing children with asthma from healthy controls, identifying poorly controlled disease, and predicting asthma exacerbation and loss of disease control. IOS, although not as readily available as spirometry, can be a useful tool in diagnosis and management of asthma in preschoolers. However, reference values for key parameters in IOS, such as AX, are still lacking, highlighting the need for further study of IOS in order to make this valuable technique more universally applicable.

FeNO is a simple noninvasive tool to measure eosinophilic airway inflammation, and levels can be used to predict response to corticosteroids. Both asthma and atopy can produce elevated FeNO. Although elevated FeNO levels have been shown to discriminate among wheezing phenotypes in infancy and school-aged children and correlate with later diagnosis of asthma diagnosis, the best use of FeNO remains unclear. FeNO levels are affected by numerous factors, and thus, interpretation of levels must be done in clinical context. FeNO levels should be viewed as easily obtainable data that, when used with other clinical and objective data, may be helpful in the diagnosis of asthma.

REFERENCES

1. National Asthma Education and Prevention Program. Expert Panel Report 3 (EPR-3): guidelines for the diagnosis and management of asthma. NIH Publication 07-4051. Bethesda (MD): National Institutes of Health; 2007.
2. 2018 GINA Report: Global Initiative for Asthma. Global strategy for asthma management and prevention 2018. Available at: www.ginasthma.com. Accessed April 24, 2018.
3. Komarow HD, Myles IA, Uzzaman A, et al. Impulse oscillometry in the evaluation of diseases of the airways in children. Ann Allergy Asthma Immunol 2011;106: 191–9.
4. Goldman MD. Clinical application of forced oscillation. Pulm Pharmacol Ther 2001;14:341–50.
5. Kattan M, Bacharier LB, O'Connor GT, et al. Spirometry and impulse oscillometry in preschool children: acceptability and relationship to maternal smoking in pregnancy. J Allergy Clin Immunol Pract 2018;6(5):1596–603.e6.

6. Batmaz SB, Kuyucu S, Arikoglu T, et al. Impulse oscillometry in acute and stable asthmatic children: a comparison with spirometry. J Asthma 2016;53:179–86.

7. Komarow HD, Skinner J, Young N, et al. Study on the use of impulse oscillometry in the evaluation of children with asthma: analysis of lung parameters, order effect, and utility compared with spirometry. Pediatr Pulmonol 2012;47:18–26.

8. Ortiz G, Menendez R. The effects of inhaled albuterol and salmeterol in 2- to 5-year-old asthmatic children as measured by impulse oscillometry. J Asthma 2002;39:531–6.

9. Nielsen KG, Bisgaard H. Discriminative capacity of bronchodilator response measured with three different lung function techniques in asthmatic and healthy children aged 2 to 5 years. Am J Respir Crit Care Med 2001;164:554–9.

10. Shi Y, Aledia AS, Tatavoosian AV, et al. Relating small airways to asthma control by using impulse oscillometry in children. J Allergy Clin Immunol 2012;129:671–8.

11. Schulze J, Biedebach S, Christmann M, et al. Impulse oscillometry as a predictor of asthma exacerbations in young children. Respiration 2016;91:107–14.

12. Shi Y, Aledia AS, Galant SP, et al. Peripheral airway impairment measured by impulse oscillometry predicts loss of asthma control in children. J Allergy Clin Immunol 2013;131:718–23.

13. Dubois AB, Botelho SY, Comroe JHA. New method for measuring airway resistance in man using a body plethysmograph: values in normal subjects and patients with respiratory disease. J Clin Invest 1956;35:327–35.

14. Smith HJ, Reinhold P, Goldman MD. Forced Oscillation Technique and Impulse Oscillometry. Lung Function Testing: European Respiratory Society Monograph. Sheffield (England): European Respiratory Society; 2005. p. 72–105.

15. Oostveen E, Boda K, van der Grinten CP, et al. Respiratory impedance in healthy subjects: baseline values and bronchodilator response. Eur Respir J 2013;42:1513–23.

16. Pride NB. Forced oscillation techniques for measuring mechanical properties of the respiratory system. Thorax 1992;47:317–20.

17. Clément J, Làndsér FJ, Van de Woestijne KP. Total resistance and reactance in patients with respiratory complaints with and without airways obstruction. Chest 1983;83:215–20.

18. Qi GS, Zhou ZC, Gu WC, et al. Detection of the airway obstruction stage in asthma using impulse oscillometry. J Asthma 2013;50:45–51.

19. Kim HY, Shin YH, Jung da W, et al. Resistance and reactance in oscillation lung function reflect basal lung function and bronchial hyperresponsiveness respectively. Respirology 2009;14:1035–41.

20. Beydon N, Davis SD, Lombardi E, et al. An official American Thoracic Society/European Respiratory Society statement: pulmonary function testing in preschool children. Am J Respir Crit Care Med 2007;175:1304–45.

21. Oostveen E, Macleod D, Lorino H, et al. The forced oscillation technique in clinical practice: methodology, recommendations and future developments. On behalf of the ERS Task Force on Respiratory Impedance Measurements. Eur Respir J 2003;22:1026–41.

22. Dencker M, Malmberg LP, Valind S, et al. Reference values for respiratory system impedance by using impulse oscillometry in children aged 2-11 years. Clin Physiol Funct Imaging 2006;26:247–50.

23. Nowowiejska B, Tomalak W, Radlinski J, et al. Transient reference values for impulse oscillometry for children aged 3-18 years. Pediatr Pulmonol 2008;43:1193–7.

24. Hellinckx J, De Boeck K, Bande-Knops J, et al. Bronchodilator response in 3-6.5 years old healthy and stable asthmatic children. Eur Respir J 1998;12:438–43.

25. Malmberg LP, Pelkonen A, Poussa T, et al. Determinants of respiratory system input impedance and bronchodilator response in healthy young Finnish preschool children. Clin Physiol Funct Imaging 2002;22:64–71.

26. Galant SP, Komarow HD, Shin H-W, et al. The case for impulse oscillometry in the management of asthma in children and adults. Ann Allergy Asthma Immunol 2017;118:664–71.

27. Frei J, Julta J, Kramer G, et al. Impulse oscillometry: reference values in children 100 to 150 cm in height and 3 to 10 years of age. Chest 2005;128:1266–73.

28. Marotta A, Klinnert MD, Price MR, et al. Impulse oscillometry provides an effective measure of lung dysfunction of 4-year-old children at risk for persistent asthma. J Allergy Clin Immunol 2003;112:317–22.

29. Knihtilä H, Kotaniemi-Syrjanen A, Pelkonen AS, et al. Sensitivity of newly defined impulse oscillometry indices in preschool children. Pediatr Pulmonol 2017;52: 598–605.

30. Nair A, Ward J, Lipworth BJ. Comparison of bronchodilator response inpatients with asthma and healthy subjects using spirometry and oscillometry. Ann Allergy Asthma Immunol 2011;107:317–22.

31. Williamson PA, Clearie K, Menzies D, et al. Assessment of small-airways disease using alveolar nitric oxide and impulse oscillometry in asthma and COPD. Lung 2011;189:121–9.

32. Song TW, Kim KW, Kim ES, et al. Utility of impulse oscillometry in young children with asthma. Pediatr Allergy Immunol 2008;19:163–8.

33. Schulze J, Smith HJ, Fuchs J, et al. Methacholine challenge in young children as evaluated by spirometry and impulse oscillometry. Respir Med 2012;106:627–34.

34. Kalliola S, Malmberg LP, Pelkonen AS, et al. Aberrant small airways function relates to asthma severity in young children. Respir Med 2016;111:16–20.

35. Knihtilä H, Kotaniemi-Syrjanen A, Makela MJ, et al. Preschool oscillometry and lung function at adolescence in asthmatic children. Pediatr Pulmonol 2015;50: 1205–13.

36. Moncada S, Higgs A. The L-arginine nitric oxide pathway. N Engl J Med 1993; 329:2002–12.

37. Dweik RA, Comhair SA, Gaston B, et al. NO chemical events in the human airway during the immediate and late antigen-induced asthmatic response. Proc Natl Acad Sci U S A 2001;98:2622–7.

38. Payne DN, Adcock IM, Wilson NM, et al. Relationship between exhaled nitric oxide and mucosal eosinophilic inflammation in children with difficult asthma after treatment with oral prednisolone. Am J Respir Crit Care Med 2001;164:1376–81.

39. Alving K, Weitzberg E, Lundberg JM. Increased amount of nitric oxide in exhaled air of asthmatics. Eur Respir J 1993;6:1368–70.

40. Sivan Y, Gadish T, Fireman E, et al. The use of exhaled nitric oxide in the diagnosis of asthma in school children. J Pediatr 2009;155:211–6.

41. Dweik RA, Boggs PB, Erzurum SC, et al. An official ATS clinical practice guideline: interpretation of exhaled nitric oxide levels (FENO) for clinical applications. Am J Respir Crit Care Med 2011;184:602–15.

42. Malinovschi A, Fonseca JA, Jacinto T, et al. Exhaled nitric oxide levels and blood eosinophil counts independently associate with wheeze and asthma events in National Health and Nutrition Examination Survey subjects. J Allergy Clin Immunol 2013;132:821–5.

43. Peirsman EJ, Carvelli TJ, Hage PY, et al. Exhaled nitric oxide in childhood allergic asthma management: a randomised controlled trial. Pediatr Pulmonol 2014;49: 624–31.
44. Ghdifan S, Verin E, Couderc L, et al. Exhaled nitric oxide fractions are well correlated with clinical control in recurrent infantile wheeze treated with inhaled corticosteroids. Pediatr Allergy Immunol 2010;21:1015–20.
45. Meyts I, Proesmans M, Van Gerven V. Tidal off-line exhaled nitric oxide measurements in a pre-school population. Eur J Pediatr 2003;162:506–10.
46. Daniel PF, Klug B, Valerius NH. Exhaled nitric oxide in healthy young children during tidal breathing through a facemask. Pediatr Allergy Immunol 2007;18:42–6.
47. van der Heijden HHACM, Brouwer ML, Hoekstra F, et al. Reference values of exhaled nitric oxide in healthy children 1-5 years using off-line tidal breathing. Pediatr Pulmonol 2014;49:291–5.
48. Jartti T, Wendelin-Saarenhovi M, Heinonen I, et al. Childhood asthma management guided by repeated FeNO measurements: a meta-analysis. Paediatr Respir Rev 2012;13:178–83.
49. Linn WS, Rappaport EB, Eckel SP, et al. Multiple-flow exhaled nitric oxide, allergy, and asthma in a population of older children. Pediatr Pulmonol 2013;48:885–96.
50. Ricciardolo FLM, Silvestri M, Pistorio A, et al. Determinants of exhaled nitric oxide levels (FeNO) in childhood atopic asthma: evidence for neonatal respiratory distress as a factor associated with low FeNO levels. J Asthma 2010;47:810–6.
51. Baraldi E, Azzolin NM, Zanconato S, et al. Corticosteroids decrease exhaled nitric oxide in children with acute asthma. J Pediatr 1997;131:381–5.
52. Pohunek P, Warner JO, Turziková J, et al. Markers of eosinophilic inflammation and tissue remodeling in children before clinically diagnosed bronchial asthma. Pediatr Allergy Immunol 2005;16:43–51.
53. Moeller A, Diefenbacher C, Lehmann A, et al. Exhaled nitric oxide distinguishes between subgroups of pre-school children with respiratory symptoms. J Allergy Clin Immunol 2008;121:705–9.
54. Balinotti JE, Colom A, Kofman C, et al. Association between the Asthma Predictive Index and levels of exhaled nitric oxide in infants and toddlers with recurrent wheezing. Arch Argent Pediatr 2013;111:191–5.
55. Debley JS, Stamey DC, Cochrane ES, et al. Exhaled nitric oxide, lung function, and exacerbations in wheezy infants and toddlers. J Allergy Clin Immunol 2010;125:1228–34.
56. Elmasri M, Romero KM, Gilman RH, et al. Longitudinal assessment of high versus low levels of fractional exhaled nitric oxide among children with asthma and atopy. Lung 2014;192:305–12.
57. Sachs-Olsen C, Lødrup Carlsen KC, Mowinckel P, et al. Diagnostic value of exhaled nitric oxide in childhood asthma and allergy. Pediatr Allergy Immunol 2010;21:e213–21.
58. Paraskaskis E, Brindicci C, Fleming L, et al. Measurement of bronchial and alveolar nitric oxide production in normal children and children with asthma. Am J Respir Crit Care Med 2006;174:260–7.
59. Caudri D, Wijga AH, Hoekstra MO, et al. Prediction of asthma in symptomatic pre-school children using exhaled nitric oxide, Rint and specific IgE. Thorax 2010;65: 801–7.
60. Singer F, Luchsinger I, Inci D, et al. Exhaled nitric oxide in symptomatic children at preschool age predicts later asthma. Allergy 2013;68:531–8.
61. Sardón O, Corcuera P, Aldasoro A, et al. Alveolar nitric oxide and its role in pediatric asthma control assessment. BMC Pulm Med 2014;14:126.

62. Gouvis-Echraghi R, Saint-Pierre P, Besharaty AA, et al. Exhaled nitric oxide measurement confirms 2 severe wheeze phenotypes in young children from the Trousseau Asthma Program. J Allergy Clin Immunol 2012;130:1005-7.
63. Van der Valk RJ, Caudri D, Savenije O, et al. Childhood wheezing phenotypes and FeNO in atopic children at age 8. Clin Exp Allergy 2012;42:1329-36.

Personalized Medicine and Pediatric Asthma

Nathan M. Pajor, MD[a], Theresa W. Guilbert, MD, MS[b,c],*

KEYWORDS

- Personalized medicine • Pediatric asthma • Biologics • Preschool • School-age
- Adolescent

KEY POINTS

- In preschool-aged children, daily inhaled corticosteroids (ICSs) are most effective in those with allergic phenotypes and more persistent symptoms, whereas intermittent therapies are effective in children with intermittent asthma, such as ICS in those with a positive modified asthma predictive index (mAPI) or azithromycin in those with a either a positive or negative mAPI.
- In school-aged children and adolescents, those with allergic phenotypes benefit most from ICSs alone or in combination with other therapies.
- Biologic therapies provide benefit to those with severe, poorly controlled, school-age children and adolescents with asthma who have eosinophilic phenotypes.
- Emerging therapies, such as macrolides and bronchial thermoplasty, and additional phenotypic markers, such as sputum inflammatory patterns, will allow for an improved, personalized approach to pediatric asthma in the future.

INTRODUCTION

Asthma is a heterogeneous disorder described by a large number of clinical features, including age of onset, triggers, atopy, frequency and severity of symptoms, and response to therapies.[1,2] Biomarkers describing the pattern of inflammation, lung function, and degree of bronchial hyperresponsiveness also help to characterize specific phenotypes.[1,2]

The existing asthma guidelines, as described previously in this journal in articles on management by Drs Kwong and Shipp, are age-based and symptom-based with the

Disclosure Statement: N.M. Pajor has no disclosures. T.W. Guilbert reports grants from NIH and Sanofi, Regeneron; personal fees from Teva, GSK, Merck, Regeneron Pharmaceuticals, Novartis/Regeneron, Sanofi/Regeneron, Aviragen, and GSK/Regneron; has consulted for American Board of Pediatrics Pediatric Pulmonary Subboard; and has royalties from UpToDate.
[a] Department of Pediatrics, Cincinnati Children's Hospital Medical Center, 3333 Burnet Avenue, MLC 7041, Cincinnati, OH 45229, USA; [b] Department of Pediatrics, University of Cincinnati, Cincinnati, OH, USA; [c] Pulmonary Division, Cincinnati Children's Hospital Medical Center, 3333 Burnet Avenue, MLC 7041, Cincinnati, OH 45229, USA
* Corresponding author. 3333 Burnet Avenue, MLC 7041, Cincinnati, OH 45229.
E-mail address: Theresa.guilbert@cchmc.org

goal of achieving adequate control through stepwise escalation of therapies.[3,4] A growing body of literature on more specific asthma phenotypes and mechanism-based endotypes provides evidence for a phenotype-based approach to management in which specific therapies are recommended based on patient and disease characteristics. This review summarizes this evidence for children ranging from preschool age to adolescence with a focus on markers of response to therapies.

PRESCHOOL
Inhaled Corticosteroids

Inhaled corticosteroids (ICSs) are first-line treatment for asthma in the preschool age group.[3,4] A recent meta-analysis emphasized their important role.[5] Looking at 3278 subjects over 15 studies, the investigators found a 30% reduction in exacerbation risk when comparing daily, medium-dose ICSs with placebo. This effect was greater in children with persistent asthma in whom a 44% risk reduction was demonstrated compared with placebo. The same meta-analysis showed a 36% reduction in exacerbations on intermittent ICS compared with placebo in intermittent asthma and when directly comparing daily and intermittent ICS showed no significant difference in the rates of exacerbation. As described in a recent review by Beigelman and Bacharier,[6] there are persistent questions about which specific phenotypes may respond more favorably to daily or intermittent ICSs. Prior analyses of children with recurrent episodic wheezing have shown that those children with Caucasian race, male sex, recent emergency department visits or hospitalizations, and aeroallergen sensitization through skin prick testing or specific immunoglobulin (Ig)E testing responded more favorably to daily ICS.[7] The INFANT (Individualized Therapy for Asthma in Toddlers) trial[8] looked at markers of treatment response through a randomized trial in which preschool-age children with mild persistent asthma received daily ICS, daily leukotriene receptor antagonist (LTRA) and intermittent, as-needed ICS. They found that greater probability of best response to daily ICS was predicted by aeroallergen sensitization and blood eosinophil counts greater than 300/μL with the greatest response observed in those participants with both features. Exacerbation history, sex, modified asthma predictive index (mAPI), serum IgE, and urinary leukotriene E4 levels did not predict a differential response.

Oral Corticosteroids

Although oral corticosteroid treatment for acute asthma exacerbation in older children and adolescents is a mainstay of therapy, extrapolation of this treatment to the preschool age group has not demonstrated the same efficacy. A meta-analysis looking at outpatients in the clinic or emergency department setting with moderate asthma or recurrent wheezing episodes showed that oral corticosteroids did not prevent hospitalizations or urgent visits and was associated with higher hospital admission rates than placebo.[9] This meta-analysis and recent Global Initiative for Asthma (GINA) guidelines[3] suggest that oral corticosteroid use should be limited in the preschool age group. However, certain subgroups of preschool children may be more likely to respond to oral corticosteroids, such as those with rhinovirus-induced wheezing or early atopic sensitization.[10]

Leukotriene Receptor Antagonists (Montelukast)

The previously described INFANT trial[8] showed that although daily ICS was most likely to be effective in children with aeroallergen sensitization and/or elevated blood eosinophil counts, alternate therapies including daily LTRA were reasonable alternatives in children without those allergic markers and showed similar effects on exacerbations. According to a recent meta-analysis, for preschoolers with episodic wheezing not stratified by allergic markers, neither daily nor intermittent LTRA led to a reduction in systemic corticosteroid courses.[11] A multicenter trial in which children age 10 months to 5 years were randomized to either montelukast or placebo did not show any clear benefit in the treatment arm but did see an increased response in those with variability in the ALOX5 gene promoter, a finding previously identified in adults.[12]

Episodic Macrolides (Azithromycin)

For children with episodic wheezing and more severe exacerbations requiring high health care utilization but minimal symptoms between episodes, azithromycin may provide significant benefit through multiple proposed mechanisms, including an anti-inflammatory effect and effects on the respiratory microbiome.[13–15] A multicenter trial[16] showed that azithromycin administration 12 mg/kg per day for 5 days started early after onset of upper respiratory tract symptoms helped to prevent progression to lower respiratory tract symptoms. The risk of progression was reduced by 36% compared with placebo, similar to the previously described improvement with ICSs. There was no difference in effect between groups with a positive or negative mAPI. Seventeen percent of those treated with azithromycin developed resistant organisms, Staphylococcus aureus most commonly, similar to 11% of those receiving placebo. Another trial[17] in preschool-age children randomized 72 children to receive either azithromycin (10 mg/kg per day for 3 days) or placebo during apparent asthma episodes and found a significant reduction of duration of symptoms (3.4 days vs 7.7 days) with a greater effect related to earlier initiation of therapy.

Summary of Preschool Age Group

As proposed in the review by Beigelman and Bacharier[6] and summarized in **Fig. 1**, a phenotypic approach to asthma management in the preschool age group would first classify children based on pattern of exacerbations and degree of impairment. Those with intermittent episodes but minimal persistent symptomatology are likely to benefit from an intermittent therapy such as ICSs or azithromycin. Oral corticosteroids have not been shown to provide clear benefit in this age group. For those with a negative mAPI, intermittent azithromycin has proven benefit in this group that has previously not been well-represented in asthma trials. Those with positive mAPI are likely to benefit from intermittent ICSs. Although there is evidence to support use of azithromycin in the positive mAPI group, there is an alternative therapy in the form of ICSs that avoids the potential risk of acquisition for azithromycin-resistant organisms. Certain clinical features (males, Caucasians, those with increased symptoms burden or health care utilization, and aeroallergen sensitization) may show increased benefit from daily ICSs. Finally, in those children with more persistent symptoms and allergic phenotypes represented by elevated eosinophils and/or aeroallergen sensitization, daily ICSs are the most effective therapy. Additional evidence and development of emerging therapies are required to better treat those children with persistent symptoms and a nonallergic phenotype.

SCHOOL-AGE CHILDREN AND ADOLESCENTS
Inhaled Corticosteroids

As in the preschool-age group, ICSs are the first-line treatment for all school-age and adolescent children with persistent asthma.[3,4] In a study of children aged 6 to 14 years with poorly controlled, mild-moderate persistent asthma, ICSs alone showed

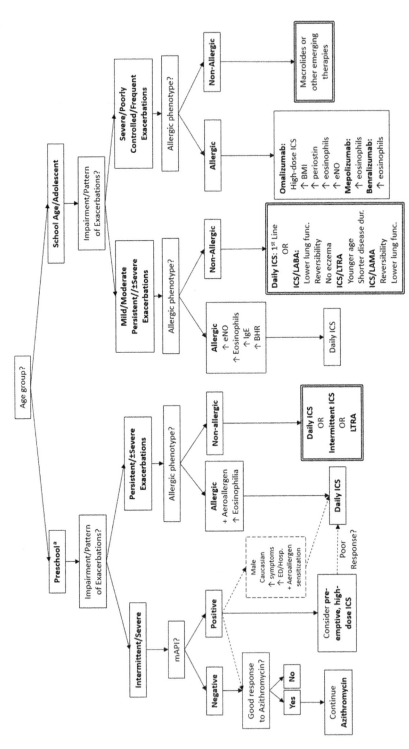

Fig. 1. Phenotype-based algorithm for management of pediatric asthma based on markers of response. [a]Limited evidence for oral corticosteroid use in the preschool age group. Double-lined box = limited evidence for treatment options in the nonallergic phenotypes. ↑, increased; BHR, bronchial hyperresponsiveness; BMI, body mass index; ED/Hosp., emergency department/hospital; eNO, exhaled nitric oxide. (*Modified from* Beigelman A, Bacharier LB. Management of preschool recurrent wheezing and asthma: a phenotype-based approach. Curr Opin Allergy Clin Immunol 2017;17(2):131–8; with permission.)

improved control over both leukotriene receptor antagonist and combination ICS/long-acting beta-agonist therapy.[18]

ICS therapy alone has shown improved control for children with the following:

1. Exhaled nitric oxide levels $\geq$25 ppb
2. Peripheral eosinophilia $\geq$5%
3. Ig E levels >150 kU/L[18,19]

A crossover study comparing ICSs with montelukast directly in children between 6 and 17 years old with mild-moderate persistent asthma showed that children with higher exhaled nitric oxide levels, total eosinophil counts, serum IgE levels, serum cationic protein levels, bronchial hyperresponsiveness on methacholine challenge, and lower baseline lung function showed a greater response in forced expiratory volume in 1 second (FEV_1) on ICSs.[20]

Oral Corticosteroids

A meta-analysis of children 3 years and older presenting to the emergency room with acute asthma symptoms demonstrated that oral corticosteroids given early in the setting of acute exacerbation reduce the need for hospitalization and remain a first-line treatment.[21] A meta-analysis of children 2 years or older with asthma ranging from mild to severe investigating early initiation of ICSs rather than systemic corticosteroids in an emergency department setting showed insufficient data to favor the use of ICSs alone.[22]

Leukotriene Receptor Antagonists (Montelukast)

In the previously described study[20] comparing ICSs with montelukast directly through a crossover design in children 6 to 17 years old with mild-moderate persistent asthma, montelukast was shown to have favorable outcomes predicted by younger age and shorter disease duration. However, another review of 2 studies in children from 2 to 14 years old with moderate symptoms has not shown significant factors predicting favorable response to montelukast.[23]

Long-Acting Beta-Agonists

Long-acting beta-agonist (LABA) therapy in combination with an ICS is a guideline-recommended step-up therapy for those with poorly controlled asthma on ICSs alone.[4] A study of children 6 to 17 years old on low-dose ICSs with mild-moderate persistent asthma who stepped-up to either medium-dose ICS, low-dose ICS/LABA, or low-dose ICS/LTRA showed significant improvement across all groups but was most significant in the LABA step-up group.[24] This response was most significant in those with lower baseline lung function. Further post hoc analysis showed that those without eczema had the most consistent improvement, whereas those without eczema had variable response depending on race and ethnicity.[25] Multiple double-blind, randomized studies examining safety with the combination of LABA and ICS therapies have helped to allay prior concerns.[26–28]

Long-Acting Muscarinic Antagonists

Tiotropium is a long-acting muscarinic antagonist (LAMA) that has been approved for children 6 years and older. When used in combination with ICSs in children with moderate to severe asthma, it has shown improved lung function and decreased symptom burden.[29,30] In adults with moderate persistent asthma, there is a greater response in those with lower baseline lung function, higher degree of bronchodilator response, and higher systemic cholinergic tone[31]; however, there currently are no data suggesting what phenotypic characteristics might predict response in children.

Biological Therapies

Omalizumab

Omalizumab is an injectable recombinant humanized IgG1 monoclonal anti-IgE antibody that can be considered in patients who are poorly controlled despite high doses of standard therapies.[32] It is approved for children 6 years or older with moderate to severe persistent asthma, evidence of perennial aeroallergen sensitivity, and inadequate control of symptoms on ICSs.[33] Injections are given every 2 to 4 weeks and there are specific IgE and weight requirements.[33] It has been shown to reduce required ICS dosing and number of exacerbations in children to moderate to severe asthma.[34,35] It has also been shown to reduce of rate of severe exacerbations, emergency department visits, hospitalizations, unscheduled office visits, rescue therapy use, and ICS dose in teenagers and adults with poorly controlled severe persistent asthma.[1,36–39] In a separate study of inner-city children with moderate to severe persistent asthma it led to improved control, reduction in seasonal peaks in exacerbations, and reduction in need for additional medications.[40] It is most effective in children and adolescents who require high-dose ICSs and experience frequent exacerbations.[41,42] A greater response has also been observed in those with higher levels of peripheral eosinophils, higher periostin (a biomarker found to correlate with T2 high inflammatory response), higher exhaled nitric oxide levels, and higher body mass index.[1,37,43–47]

Mepolizumab

Mepolizumab is a humanized monoclonal antibody against interleukin (IL)-5 aimed at those with severe eosinophilic asthma.[32,48] It is approved for children older than 12 years as an add-on therapy in those with severe persistent asthma and an eosinophilic phenotype, and it is given subcutaneously every 4 weeks.[49] It has been showed to increase FEV_1, reduce exacerbations requiring emergency room visits and hospitalizations, and improve control and symptoms.[50,51] Greater response is related to higher blood eosinophil levels.[50,51]

Benralizumab

Benralizumab is a humanized monoclonal antibody targeting the alpha subunit of the IL-5 receptor, also aimed at those with severe and poorly controlled eosinophilic asthma.[32,52] It has been showed to reduce oral glucocorticoid needs and exacerbation rates.[53] It was recently approved as an add-on maintenance therapy for children age 12 and older with severe asthma and eosinophilic phenotype, and it is given subcutaneously at 4-week intervals for the first 3 doses and then every 8 weeks.[54]

Emerging Therapies

There are a limited number of studies of children with nonallergic, typically neutrophil predominant, phenotypes. Chronic azithromycin is often used in cystic fibrosis for neutrophilic inflammation. Meta-analysis of azithromycin in adults with severe asthma did not show significant benefit above placebo; however, 2 of the included studies did show possible benefit in noneosinophilic asthma.[55] A recent randomized, placebo-controlled, double-blinded study in adults with persistent asthma requiring ICSs and long-acting bronchodilators showed that azithromycin treatment resulted in fewer asthma exacerbations and improved quality of life in both eosinophilic and noneosinophilic asthma.[56] Additional research is needed in the school-age pediatric age group.

Bronchial thermoplasty is a radiofrequency-generated thermal treatment of the airways by flexible bronchoscopy intended to reduce airway smooth muscle mass.[57]

Treatment has been shown to reduce severe exacerbations and reduce emergency department visits in adults with severe, uncontrolled asthma.[58,59] This treatment is currently approved only for those 18 years and older and there have been no studies in the pediatric or adolescent age groups.[60]

Several studies have looked at additional phenotypic markers that may be useful in the future for stratifying and further tailoring treatment of children with severe asthma. One recent cohort trial of individuals 6 to 18 years old with severe asthma had a number of inflammatory markers followed over a 3-month period. Comparisons between those who were treatment-refractory and those who achieved control showed that sputum neutrophils, IL-10, interferon-γ, tumor necrosis factor-α, and granulocyte-macrophage colony-stimulating factor were higher in the refractory group.[61] There was no difference seen in fractional exhaled nitric oxide (FeNO) in this study. Prior meta-analyses combining adult and pediatric data across a range of asthma severities using both FeNO and sputum eosinophils to dictate medical management showed that likelihood of exacerbations decreased but asthma control based on symptom score and lung function were not impacted.[62]

Other Considerations for Adolescents

Management of chronic illness in the adolescent population presents unique challenges that differ from the younger, school-age child. A range of environmental, psychosocial, behavioral, and lifestyle factors impact asthma control in this age group.[63–65] It is important that providers consider these factors when choosing therapies. Multiple studies[66–68] have shown that incorporating psychosocial interventions through behavioral and cognitive-behavioral approaches in combination with education about the disease and medications has resulted in improved medication adherence, reduced asthma severity, and reduced psychological problems that have been described in association with severe asthma.

Summary of School-Age and Adolescent Age Group

For school-age and adolescent children with mild persistent asthma who have an allergic phenotype marked by elevated eosinophils and elevated IgE levels in addition to increased bronchial hyperresponsiveness and higher levels of exhaled nitric oxide, ICSs remain the first-line treatment, whereas leukotriene receptor antagonists can be considered as first-line treatment in children of younger age or shorter disease duration. Step-up therapies, such as leukotriene receptor antagonists, LABAs and LAMAs, in combination with ICSs have all been shown to have benefit, with ICS/LABA showing greater efficacy than ICS/LTRA, especially in those with lower baseline lung function and in those without eczema. Specific evidence for how ICS/LAMA combinations perform for specific phenotypes and in comparison with other combinations is not yet available in the pediatric age range. For children with severe asthma, frequent or severe exacerbations, and poor control on the therapies described previously, multiple biologic agents are available. All have shown to be more beneficial in children with higher eosinophil levels and omalizumab has been shown to have greater efficacy in those with poor control on high-dose ICSs, higher exhaled nitric oxide levels, higher periostin, and higher body-mass index. Current Food and Drug Administration approvals regarding age range and dosing regimens must be taken into account when tailoring biologic therapy to a specific patient. For children with nonallergic phenotypes, there is less evidence guiding phenotype-specific therapy. Finally, although important in all patients, addressing psychosocial, environmental, behavioral, and lifestyle factors in the adolescent population is crucial to establishing improved asthma control.

SUMMARY

The optimal treatment strategy for a child with asthma is not yet clearly defined. An increase in the number of available therapies for children with asthma coupled with a growing body of evidence on specific phenotypes within this heterogeneous disease suggest a phenotype-based approach will allow for improved asthma management. The evidence reviewed is limited in children and often based on post hoc analyses, so should be regarded as preliminary. Improved understanding of specific asthma phenotypes and research into targeted therapies is likely to significantly improve asthma treatment in the future.

REFERENCES

1. Mokhallati N, Guilbert TW. Moving towards precision care for childhood asthma. Curr Opin Pediatr 2016;28(3):331–8.
2. Cowan K, Guilbert TW. Pediatric asthma phenotypes. Curr Opin Pediatr 2012; 24(3):344–51.
3. From the global strategy for asthma management and prevention. Global initiative for asthma (GINA). 2018.
4. National Asthma Education and Prevention Program. Expert Panel Report 3 (EPR-3): guidelines for the diagnosis and management of asthma—summary report 2007. J Allergy Clin Immunol 2007;120(5 Suppl):S94–138.
5. Kaiser SV, Huynh T, Bacharier LB, et al. Preventing exacerbations in preschoolers with recurrent wheeze: a meta-analysis. Pediatrics 2016;137(6) [pii:e20154496].
6. Beigelman A, Bacharier LB. Management of preschool recurrent wheezing and asthma: a phenotype-based approach. Curr Opin Allergy Clin Immunol 2017; 17(2):131–8.
7. Bacharier LB, Guilbert TW, Zeiger RS, et al. Patient characteristics associated with improved outcomes with use of an inhaled corticosteroid in preschool children at risk for asthma. J Allergy Clin Immunol 2009;123(5):1077–82, 1082.e1-5.
8. Fitzpatrick AM, Jackson DJ, Mauger DT, et al. Individualized therapy for persistent asthma in young children. J Allergy Clin Immunol 2016;138(6):1608–18.e12.
9. Castro-Rodriguez JA, Beckhaus AA, Forno E. Efficacy of oral corticosteroids in the treatment of acute wheezing episodes in asthmatic preschoolers: systematic review with meta-analysis. Pediatr Pulmonol 2016;51(8):868–76.
10. Beigelman A, Durrani S, Guilbert TW. Should a preschool child with acute episodic wheeze be treated with oral corticosteroids? A Pro/Con debate. J Allergy Clin Immunol Pract 2016;4(1):27–35.
11. Brodlie M, Gupta A, Rodriguez-Martinez CE, et al. Leukotriene receptor antagonists as maintenance and intermittent therapy for episodic viral wheeze in children. Cochrane Database Syst Rev 2015;(10):CD008202.
12. Nwokoro C, Pandya H, Turner S, et al. Intermittent montelukast in children aged 10 months to 5 years with wheeze (WAIT trial): a multicentre, randomised, placebo-controlled trial. Lancet Respir Med 2014;2(10):796–803.
13. Beigelman A, Isaacson-Schmid M, Sajol G, et al. Randomized trial to evaluate azithromycin's effects on serum and upper airway IL-8 levels and recurrent wheezing in infants with respiratory syncytial virus bronchiolitis. J Allergy Clin Immunol 2015;135(5):1171–8.e1.
14. Beigelman A, Mikols CL, Gunsten SP, et al. Azithromycin attenuates airway inflammation in a mouse model of viral bronchiolitis. Respir Res 2010;11:90.
15. Zhou Y, Bacharier LB, Isaacson-Schmid M, et al. Azithromycin therapy during respiratory syncytial virus bronchiolitis: upper airway microbiome alterations

and subsequent recurrent wheeze. J Allergy Clin Immunol 2016;138(4): 1215–9.e5.

16. Bacharier LB, Guilbert TW, Mauger DT, et al. Early administration of azithromycin and prevention of severe lower respiratory tract illnesses in preschool children with a history of such illnesses: a randomized clinical trial. JAMA 2015;314(19): 2034–44.

17. Stokholm J, Chawes BL, Vissing NH, et al. Azithromycin for episodes with asthma-like symptoms in young children aged 1-3 years: a randomised, double-blind, placebo-controlled trial. Lancet Respir Med 2016;4(1):19–26.

18. Sorkness CA, Lemanske RF Jr, Mauger DT, et al. Long-term comparison of 3 controller regimens for mild-moderate persistent childhood asthma: the Pediatric Asthma Controller Trial. J Allergy Clin Immunol 2007;119(1):64–72.

19. Knuffman JE, Sorkness CA, Lemanske RF Jr, et al. Phenotypic predictors of long-term response to inhaled corticosteroid and leukotriene modifier therapies in pediatric asthma. J Allergy Clin Immunol 2009;123(2):411–6.

20. Szefler SJ, Phillips BR, Martinez FD, et al. Characterization of within-subject responses to fluticasone and montelukast in childhood asthma. J Allergy Clin Immunol 2005;115(2):233–42.

21. Rowe BH, Spooner C, Ducharme FM, et al. Early emergency department treatment of acute asthma with systemic corticosteroids. Cochrane Database Syst Rev 2001;(1):CD002178.

22. Edmonds ML, Camargo CA Jr, Pollack CV Jr, et al. Early use of inhaled corticosteroids in the emergency department treatment of acute asthma. Cochrane Database Syst Rev 2003;(3):CD002308.

23. Meyer KA, Arduino JM, Santanello NC, et al. Response to montelukast among subgroups of children aged 2 to 14 years with asthma. J Allergy Clin Immunol 2003;111(4):757–62.

24. Lemanske RF Jr, Mauger DT, Sorkness CA, et al. Step-up therapy for children with uncontrolled asthma receiving inhaled corticosteroids. N Engl J Med 2010; 362(11):975–85.

25. Malka J, Mauger DT, Covar R, et al. Eczema and race as combined determinants for differential response to step-up asthma therapy. J Allergy Clin Immunol 2014; 134(2):483–5.

26. Stempel DA, Raphiou IH, Kral KM, et al. Serious asthma events with fluticasone plus salmeterol versus fluticasone alone. N Engl J Med 2016;374(19):1822–30.

27. Stempel DA, Szefler SJ, Pedersen S, et al. Safety of adding salmeterol to fluticasone propionate in children with asthma. N Engl J Med 2016;375(9):840–9.

28. Peters SP, Bleecker ER, Canonica GW, et al. Serious asthma events with budesonide plus formoterol vs. budesonide alone. N Engl J Med 2016;375(9):850–60.

29. Hamelmann E, Bateman ED, Vogelberg C, et al. Tiotropium add-on therapy in adolescents with moderate asthma: a 1-year randomized controlled trial. J Allergy Clin Immunol 2016;138(2):441–50.e8.

30. Rodrigo GJ, Castro-Rodríguez JA. Tiotropium for the treatment of adolescents with moderate to severe symptomatic asthma: a systematic review with meta-analysis. Ann Allergy Asthma Immunol 2015;115(3):211–6.

31. Peters SP, Bleecker ER, Kunselman SJ, et al. Predictors of response to tiotropium versus salmeterol in asthmatic adults. J Allergy Clin Immunol 2013;132(5): 1068–74.e1.

32. Burg GT, Covar R, Oland AA, et al. The tempest: difficult to control asthma in adolescence. J Allergy Clin Immunol Pract 2018;6(3):738–48.

33. Omalizumab FDA Label. Food and drug administration. Available at: www. accessdata.fda.gov/drugsatfda_docs/label/2016/103976s5225lbl.pdf. Accessed February 8, 2018.
34. Lemanske RF Jr, Nayak A, McAlary M, et al. Omalizumab improves asthma-related quality of life in children with allergic asthma. Pediatrics 2002;110(5):e55.
35. Milgrom H, Berger W, Nayak A, et al. Treatment of childhood asthma with anti-immunoglobulin E antibody (omalizumab). Pediatrics 2001;108(2):E36.
36. Bousquet J, Cabrera P, Berkman N, et al. The effect of treatment with omalizumab, an anti-IgE antibody, on asthma exacerbations and emergency medical visits in patients with severe persistent asthma. Allergy 2005;60(3):302–8.
37. Hanania NA, Alpan O, Hamilos DL, et al. Omalizumab in severe allergic asthma inadequately controlled with standard therapy: a randomized trial. Ann Intern Med 2011;154(9):573–82.
38. Holgate ST, Chuchalin AG, Hébert J, et al. Efficacy and safety of a recombinant anti-immunoglobulin E antibody (omalizumab) in severe allergic asthma. Clin Exp Allergy 2004;34(4):632–8.
39. Humbert M, Beasley R, Ayres J, et al. Benefits of omalizumab as add-on therapy in patients with severe persistent asthma who are inadequately controlled despite best available therapy (GINA 2002 step 4 treatment): INNOVATE. Allergy 2005; 60(3):309–16.
40. Busse WW, Morgan WJ, Gergen PJ, et al. Randomized trial of omalizumab (anti-IgE) for asthma in inner-city children. N Engl J Med 2011;364(11):1005–15.
41. Brodlie M, McKean MC, Moss S, et al. The oral corticosteroid-sparing effect of omalizumab in children with severe asthma. Arch Dis Child 2012;97(7):604–9.
42. Lanier B, Bridges T, Kulus M, et al. Omalizumab for the treatment of exacerbations in children with inadequately controlled allergic (IgE-mediated) asthma. J Allergy Clin Immunol 2009;124(6):1210–6.
43. Guilbert TW, Bacharier LB, Fitzpatrick AM. Severe asthma in children. J Allergy Clin Immunol Pract 2014;2(5):489–500.
44. Hanania NA, Wenzel S, Rosén K, et al. Exploring the effects of omalizumab in allergic asthma: an analysis of biomarkers in the EXTRA study. Am J Respir Crit Care Med 2013;187(8):804–11.
45. Fajt ML, Wenzel SE. Asthma phenotypes and the use of biologic medications in asthma and allergic disease: the next steps toward personalized care. J Allergy Clin Immunol 2015;135(2):299–310 [quiz: 311].
46. Sorkness CA, Wildfire JJ, Calatroni A, et al. Reassessment of omalizumab-dosing strategies and pharmacodynamics in inner-city children and adolescents. J Allergy Clin Immunol Pract 2013;1(2):163–71.
47. Busse W, Spector S, Rosén K, et al. High eosinophil count: a potential biomarker for assessing successful omalizumab treatment effects. J Allergy Clin Immunol 2013;132(2):485–6.e11.
48. Bel EH, Wenzel SE, Thompson PJ, et al. Oral glucocorticoid-sparing effect of mepolizumab in eosinophilic asthma. N Engl J Med 2014;371(13):1189–97.
49. Mepolizumab FDA Label. Food and drug administration. Available at: www. accessdata.fda.gov/drugsatfda_docs/label/2015/125526orig1s000lbl.pdf.
50. Ortega HG, Liu MC, Pavord ID, et al. Mepolizumab treatment in patients with severe eosinophilic asthma. N Engl J Med 2014;371(13):1198–207.
51. Pavord ID, Korn S, Howarth P, et al. Mepolizumab for severe eosinophilic asthma (DREAM): a multicentre, double-blind, placebo-controlled trial. Lancet 2012; 380(9842):651–9.

52. Nair P, Wenzel S, Rabe KF, et al. Oral glucocorticoid-sparing effect of benralizu-mab in severe asthma. N Engl J Med 2017;376(25):2448–58.
53. FitzGerald JM, Bleecker ER, Menzies-Gow A, et al. Predictors of enhanced response with benralizumab for patients with severe asthma: pooled analysis of the SIROCCO and CALIMA studies. Lancet Respir Med 2018;6(1):51–64.
54. Benralizumab FDA Label. Food and drug administration. Available at: www.accessdata.fda.gov/drugsatfda_docs/label/2017/761070s000lbl.pdf.
55. Kew KM, Undela K, Kotortsi I, et al. Macrolides for chronic asthma. Cochrane Database Syst Rev 2015;(9):CD002997.
56. Gibson PG, Yang IA, Upham JW, et al. Effect of azithromycin on asthma exacer-bations and quality of life in adults with persistent uncontrolled asthma (AMAZES): a randomised, double-blind, placebo-controlled trial. Lancet 2017; 390(10095):659–68.
57. Blaiss MS, Castro M, Chipps BE, et al. Guiding principles for use of newer bio-logics and bronchial thermoplasty for patients with severe asthma. Ann Allergy Asthma Immunol 2017;119(6):533–40.
58. Castro M, Rubin AS, Laviolette M, et al. Effectiveness and safety of bronchial ther-moplasty in the treatment of severe asthma: a multicenter, randomized, double-blind, sham-controlled clinical trial. Am J Respir Crit Care Med 2010;181(2): 116–24.
59. Wechsler ME, Laviolette M, Rubin AS, et al. Bronchial thermoplasty: long-term safety and effectiveness in patients with severe persistent asthma. J Allergy Clin Immunol 2013;132(6):1295–302.
60. Peters SP, Busse WW. New and anticipated therapies for severe asthma. J Allergy Clin Immunol Pract 2017;5(5S):S15–24.
61. Eller MCN, Vergani KP, Saraiva-Romanholo BM, et al. Can inflammatory markers in induced sputum be used to detect phenotypes and endotypes of pediatric se-vere therapy-resistant asthma? Pediatr Pulmonol 2018;53(9):1208–17.
62. Petsky HL, Cates CJ, Kew KM, et al. Tailoring asthma treatment on eosinophilic markers (exhaled nitric oxide or sputum eosinophils): a systematic review and meta-analysis. Thorax 2018;73(12):1110–9.
63. Fitzpatrick AM. Severe asthma in children: lessons learned and future directions. J Allergy Clin Immunol Pract 2016;4(1):11–9 [quiz: 20–1].
64. Oland AA, Booster GD, Bender BG. Psychological and lifestyle risk factors for asthma exacerbations and morbidity in children. World Allergy Organ J 2017; 10(1):35.
65. Oren E, Gerald L, Stern DA, et al. Self-reported stressful life events during adoles-cence and subsequent asthma: a longitudinal study. J Allergy Clin Immunol Pract 2017;5(2):427–34.e2.
66. Chen SH, Huang JL, Yeh KW, et al. Interactive support interventions for care-givers of asthmatic children. J Asthma 2013;50(6):649–57.
67. Duncan CL, Hogan MB, Tien KJ, et al. Efficacy of a parent-youth teamwork inter-vention to promote adherence in pediatric asthma. J Pediatr Psychol 2013;38(6): 617–28.
68. Long KA, Ewing LJ, Cohen S, et al. Preliminary evidence for the feasibility of a stress management intervention for 7- to 12-year-olds with asthma. J Asthma 2011;48(2):162–70.

Treatment Adherence in Young Children with Asthma

Genery D. Booster, PhD*, Alyssa A. Oland, PhD, Bruce G. Bender, PhD

KEYWORDS

- Children • Asthma • Adherence • Intervention

KEY POINTS

- Treatment adherence in young children involves multiple, bidirectional factors including the child, family, community, and health care system.
- Effective interventions to promote treatment adherence involve multiple components including monitoring, feedback, education, and cognitive/behavioral interventions.
- Additional research is needed to identify essential treatment components, address potential developmental factors, and promote sustainment of intervention effects.

INTRODUCTION

An estimated 6.8 million children in the United States are affected by asthma,[1] which places them at significant risk for hospitalizations, emergency room visits, and school absences.[2–4] Although inhaled corticosteroids (ICS) have long been identified as important and effective medications in the prevention of asthma attacks, improving asthma control,[5,6] and reducing asthma morbidity and mortality,[7,8] research has repeatedly shown that adherence to these medications is low.[8,9] For young children, studies have found adherence rates frequently below 50%.[10] Pediatric patients and their parents may also have difficulty following asthma management recommendations, such as identification and avoidance of triggers and engagement in physical activities.[11] As a result, many children experience illness exacerbations with significant effects on their quality of life[5,12] and health[13] that could otherwise have been avoided.

Self-management in chronic illness has traditionally been defined by the US Institute of Medicine as "the tasks that individuals must undertake to live with one or more chronic conditions. These tasks include having the confidence to deal with medical management, role management, and emotional management of their conditions."[14] For young children, however, this definition may not take into account the complex conditions that are a part of managing illness within a family environment. In an effort

Disclosure Statement: The authors do not have anything to disclose.
National Jewish Health, Pediatric Behavioral Health, 1400 Jackson Street, Denver, CO 80206, USA
* Corresponding author.
E-mail address: boosterg@njhealth.org

to capture the ecological factors present in a young child's life, Modi and colleagues[15] have developed a comprehensive framework to conceptualize self-management in pediatric populations. The Pediatric Self-Management Model[15] defines self-management as "the interaction of health behaviors and related processes that patients and families engage in to care for a chronic condition."[15] From this ecological perspective, bidirectional self-management processes occur within the domains of the child, the family, the community, and the health care system. This conceptualization is consistent with recent research, framing child asthma management as a shared process that occurs between a child, his or her caregivers, and his or her medical provider(s).[16]

MODIFIABLE FACTORS RELATED TO TREATMENT NONADHERENCE

Although recent research has provided substantial information regarding factors related to treatment adherence in children, most studies have focused on older children and adolescents.[4,17,18] Among young children (ie, birth through 8 years), research suggests adherence may be related to several factors within the child, family, community, and health care system domains (**Table 1**).

Individual and Family Factors

Within the context of the individual, children's behaviors and characteristics have been associated with differences in treatment adherence. For young children, factors such

Table 1		
Ecological model of intervention for young children with asthma		
Domain	**Modifiable Targets**	**Interventions**
Individual	Child beliefs about medication Child's emotional and behavioral functioning Child's organizational skills Child's understanding of asthma and medications	Asthma education programs Behavioral and incentive programs (positive reinforcement, rewards, and token reinforcement) Motivational interventions Self-monitoring interventions
Family	Parent beliefs about medication Parent's emotional and behavioral functioning Parent's organizational skills Parenting skills and confidence Parent's understanding of asthma management and medications	Asthma education programs Behavioral and incentive programs Motivational interventions Parent management training Tailoring treatment regimen to patient's lifestyle, such as taking medications with meals Positive parenting programs
Community	Access to medications and interventions at school Bullying and peer relationships Relationships with teachers and teacher understanding of asthma management	School-based intervention programs 504 and asthma action plans School-based positive behavior support programs
Health care system	Access to medications and health care providers Communication between patients, families, and health care providers Financial and insurance supports	Interventions aimed at improving the treatment alliance between families and health care providers Telemedicine opportunities Health care provider communication and feedback regarding patient adherence

as oppositional behaviors,[19] cognitive capacity,[16,19] emotional functioning,[16,19] and development[6] have been linked to differences in adherence to medications. Resistant and noncompliant behaviors in young children often result in poor treatment adherence, as parents may be unable to administer breathing treatments (eg, keeping a facemask on an infant or active toddler[6]). Among parents of children between 18 months and 7 years, a child's reaction to being given medication was identified as one of the most common reasons for missing administration of controller medications.[20] Parents and caregivers of children with chronic illness frequently report challenges with their child's treatment routines, and children with asthma have been shown to display more behavioral challenges than their healthy peers.[21,22] Parents of children with asthma may have increased difficulty effectively managing developmentally appropriate challenges such as temper tantrums, out of concern that crying behaviors may trigger breathing difficulties.[22] Giving in to these negative behaviors, however, may increase tantrums and conflict[23] and may lead to more oppositional behaviors during treatment regimens.[11] Similarly, psychosocial factors such as anxiety, attention capacity, and hyperactive behaviors have been associated with changes in symptom perception,[16,23,24] which, in turn, may affect use of rescue medications. One study examining older children (ages 8–12 years) found preliminary evidence that dispositional hope (having a belief in one's ability to achieve one's goals and overcome barriers) was a significant predictor of adherence of medication adherence, beyond forced expiratory volume in 1 second (FEV_1).[25] To the best of the authors' knowledge, however, this individual factor has not been examined in younger children.

Young children rely on caregivers for access to and administration of asthma medications and for implementing environmental controls, such as a home environment free of tobacco smoke.[26] For young children, factors that can contribute to medication nonadherence include lack of access to medications,[27] parental concerns regarding the cost of medications,[28] improper inhaler technique,[27] and parents forgetting to give their children inhaled corticosteroids.[20] Parents who have poor knowledge of asthma and asthma medications[29,30] and are fearful of possible negative effects from inhaled corticosteroids[28,30] are less likely to give their children prescribed inhaled corticosteroids. Interviews with parents of children with asthma revealed concerns with medication adverse effects or dependency that undermined treatment adherence.[31] Parents may intentionally choose to not administer medications to their children, for example, believing they are acting in their child's best interest because of a lack of understanding and/or fears regarding the asthma medication. Additionally, parents may have difficulty identifying and avoiding environmental triggers[11] and may not accurately recognize their child's symptoms,[29] which can lead to poorer asthma management.

For caregivers, the experience of parenting a young child with asthma can be stressful, particularly as evidence suggests that children with asthma experience more emotional[32] and behavioral challenges[33] than their healthy peers. Parents of children with asthma have also been shown to have significant emotional challenges,[34] including increased depression[31] and anxiety.[35] As such, these parents may have fewer internal resources for managing the increased parental demands placed by children with asthma and co-occurring emotional and/or behavioral issues. Accordingly, parental emotional distress and parenting stress are associated with increased use of smoking tobacco in the home, poorer inhaler technique,[36] more difficulty completing daily asthma management tasks,[37] and increased treatment nonadherence.[20,36,38]

Further, parents experiencing psychological distress tend to have lower confidence in their abilities,[39] be more critical with their children,[40] have more parenting difficulties, and have a more strained parent-child relationship.[41] These factors are also associated with poorer adherence and increased disease severity. Additionally, parental noninvolvement is associated with nonadherence,[42] and parents who are experiencing psychological distress and/or parenting stress may be at particular risk for reduced involvement with their children. These children, in turn, may spend more time in sedentary activities, such as time on electronics, which is associated with increased asthma morbidity.[43] In this manner, there seems to be a reciprocal pattern, whereby child problems, parent psychological distress, issues in the parent-child relationship, parenting difficulties, and problems with completion of asthma management tasks contribute to and exacerbate each other.[11]

Community and Systems-Related Factors

In order for children and families to adhere to medical recommendations, they must have appropriate medical care and follow-up. Research suggests that children living in poverty, both in urban and rural communities, are more likely not to receive preventative medications and appropriate follow up care[44–46] and are at increased risk for treatment nonadherence.[4] Poor communication or conflict between parents and health care providers has also been associated with treatment nonadherence.[47] Even when families do have appropriate communication with providers and receive asthma action plans, these plans are usually written at a seventh to ninth grade reading level, which may present challenges for families with fewer educational opportunities.[48] Children with asthma living in rural areas may experience additional barriers to health care, such as travel requirements and a lack of local providers.[49]

Children from low-income, urban households have also been shown to receive poorer quality of treatment,[50] have increased exposure to polluted air and water,[51] and have increased exposure to tobacco smoke and pollutants.[52] They have also been shown to have increased exposure to environmental stressors, such as dangerous neighborhoods,[53,54] housing-related stress,[51] family conflict,[53] and chronic family stress.[55] It is believed that this exposure to chronic environmental stressors can exacerbate asthma through heightening a child's inflammatory profile[56] and by contributing to parental stress, which, in turn, can contribute to treatment nonadherence.[20,36,38] Further, children from low-income urban families may have reduced parental support and involvement[51] and may spend more time watching television,[53] which can further contribute to difficulties with asthma management. In short, numerous life challenges and sources of stress may undermine a family's resources and capacity to manage childhood asthma, including adhering to a treatment plan.

Although psychosocial interventions are unlikely to directly affect a child's socioeconomic status, community resources can be effectively leveraged to moderate this risk factor. Improving access to medications at school and providing controller medications at school may reduce barriers to treatment adherence in at-risk communities.[4] In contrast, other community factors such as peer influence and perceptions may decrease medication adherence. Evidence suggests that some children may feel embarrassed when taking medications at school, which may lead to poorer adherence to medications.[4] Research has also found lower levels of treatment adherence among parents experiencing a lack of community support.[29]

INTERVENTIONS TO PROMOTE TREATMENT ADHERENCE

As discussed previously, the Pediatric Self-Management Model[15] identifies clear areas for intervention at the individual, family, community, and system levels.

Psychosocial interventions aimed at improving adherence have traditionally included educational components (eg, education about asthma, triggers, medication, peak flows, and inhaler technique), creation of an asthma action plan, and behavioral techniques such as self-management strategies, feedback, and incentive plans.[4] Although most studies have been conducted with older children, preliminary research suggests that such techniques may be effective for young children also.[57,58] Patient advocates, medical assistants who help low income adults with asthma to navigate health care systems and follow their treatment plan, can improve adherence and disease control in adults[59] and children.[60] Similarly, community health workers, volunteers who often share the culture with patients in safety-net practices, can also play an important role in keeping families engaged with their health care provider and treatment plan.[61]

Asthma education and adherence monitoring have long been used to promote treatment adherence among individuals with asthma,[62] and there is evidence to suggest that simply monitoring and providing feedback to parents about adherence levels may lead to improvements in treatment adherence for young children. One recent study, for example, found that simply asking parents to bring in medication canisters for weighing at doctor's appointments resulted in increases in treatment adherence and fewer asthma exacerbations when compared with previous research.[63] Additional recent studies with children ages 6 to 17 suggest that asthma education with use of electronic monitoring devices, Web-based interactive communication programs, and feedback from health care providers may improve treatment adherence and reduce asthma symptoms.[58,64–67] Importantly, research from Spaulding and colleagues[64] suggests that feedback from health care providers may be a key component of such interventions, as results from their single-subject design study revealed that adherence became more variable once feedback was withdrawn. Although this study is limited by its small sample size, future research in this area is warranted.

Despite these positive effects, investigations suggest that interventions that include behavioral and cognitive strategies, in addition to patient education, may be the most effective in improving treatment adherence and patient outcomes.[68] Various cognitive behavioral and multicomponent interventions have been developed for young children with asthma. A meta-analysis examining psychological interventions aimed at promoting treatment adherence in children with chronic health conditions suggested that such interventions demonstrate medium effect sizes, compared with small effect sizes found for educational interventions alone.[18] Although a more recent meta-analysis[17] found smaller effect sizes for interventions published between 2008 and 2013, the authors note these studies were limited by methodological challenges. An examination of studies aimed specifically at young children with asthma suggests that cognitive behavioral strategies such as contingency management, token reinforcement, goal setting, and problem-solving skills training may improve treatment adherence and reduce asthma exacerbations.[57,69–71] However, 1 study reported that adherence benefits may not be maintained once behavioral incentives are removed.[70]

In addition to interventions that focus on traditional targets such as asthma-related behaviors and compliance with treatment regimens, emerging research suggests that parenting interventions may be an important adjunct to these interventions for parents of young children with asthma. Morawska and colleagues (2016),[72] for example, have applied positive parenting strategies to families of children with asthma. This intervention included 2 interactive group sessions that focused on strategies to empower parents to prevent and manage behavior problems, implement asthma treatment plans, promote a positive parent-child relationship, and utilize effective discipline strategies. Results indicate that children of parents who received the positive parenting intervention had significantly fewer asthma episodes and greater improvement in parent-reported family quality of life than those who received care as usual.

Interventions at the community and system levels have also been developed to promote treatment adherence in young children. Two recent studies suggest that utilizing school resources and telemedicine opportunities may improve adherence and asthma outcomes.[73,74] For example, 1 group found that use of a school-based telemedicine program that involved supervised medication administration at school combined with telemedicine family follow-up resulted in more symptom-free days and fewer emergency room visits when compared with students who did not receive this intervention.[73] For children at high risk for asthma exacerbations and treatment nonadherence, such as those from urban, rural, and low-income communities, utilizing community resources and novel health care technology may be especially helpful.

LIMITATIONS AND FUTURE DIRECTIONS

Despite the promising research discussed previously, results are limited by several methodological challenges including small sample sizes, lack of control groups in some studies, inconsistent measurement of treatment adherence, a lack of developmentally specific interventions, and wide age ranges included in most studies.[17] As a result, it is difficult to determine whether the interventions were effective and appropriate for all age groups. Additionally, few studies have developed interventions for young children in high-risk communities, and none have examined which intervention components may be most effective or essential.

Although research suggests that adolescents are at highest risk for challenges with adherence,[75] relatively few studies have examined challenges that may be particular to families with young children.[4] Most studies looking at interventions for children with asthma have included patients across childhood and adolescence and have not examined developmental effects or impact.[17,18] It is possible that particular interventions may be more appropriate for certain age levels, or that developmental factors may affect treatment delivery and impact. Future research should investigate the impact of child development on treatment effectiveness and treatment adherence.

Further, to the best of the authors' knowledge, no research to date has focused on the development of adherence interventions that are specifically tailored to community needs. Although a growing body of literature has carefully examined barriers to treatment adherence,[19] little research has directly linked intervention targets to identified barriers within a specific community or examined interventions related to changing the peer communities. Findings from community-based participatory research (CBPR) suggest that the inclusion of stakeholder input (ie, from parents, children, health care providers, and community leaders) increases feasibility of implementation, stakeholder buy-in, and intervention sustainment.[76,77] This may be especially important for high-risk communities, as some research suggests that short-term improvements in adherence may not be maintained over time.[57]

In summary, treatment nonadherence in young children with asthma involves multiple factors and should be viewed within an ecological framework. Few interventions have targeted multiple bidirectional factors, however, and little research has examined which interventions may be most appropriate for young children. Additional research is needed to identify essential intervention components and to determine how to sustain such interventions in at-risk communities. Pediatric psychologists, with training in psychosocial intervention, screening, and primary prevention models may be uniquely equipped to partner with communities and medical settings to develop and sustain targeted interventions for young children with asthma.

REFERENCES

1. Bloom BC, Cohen RA. Summary health statistics for U.S. children: national health interview survey, 2006. Hyattsville (MD): National Center for Health Statistics; 2007.

2. Chipps BE, Zeiger RS, Borish L, et al, TENOR Study Group. Key findings and clinical implications from the epidemiology and natural history of asthma: Outcomes and treatment regiments (TENOR) study. J Allergy Clin Immunol 2012; 130:332–42.e10.

3. Liu AH, Gilsenan AW, Stanford RH, et al. Status of asthma control in pediatric primary care: Results from the pediatric asthma control characteristics and prevalence survey study (ACESS). J Pediatr 2010;157:276–81.e3.

4. Gray WN, Netz M, McConville A, et al. Medication adherence in pediatric asthma: a systematic review of the literature. Pediatr Pulmonol 2018;53:668–84.

5. National Asthma Education Prevention Program (NAEPP). Expert panel report 3 (EPR-3): guidelines for the diagnosis and management of asthma-summary report 2007. J Allergy Clin Immunol 2007;120(5 Suppl):S94–138.

6. Blake KV. Improving adherence to asthma medications: current knowledge and future perspectives. Curr Opin Pulm Med 2017;23:62–70.

7. Bauman LJ, Wright E, Leickly EE, et al. Relationship of adherence to pediatric asthma morbidity among inner-city children. Pediatrics 2002;110:e1–7.

8. McQuaid EL, Kopel SJ, Klein RB, et al. Medication adherence in pediatric asthma: reasoning, responsibility, and behavior. J Pediatr Psychol 2003;28: 323–33.

9. Bender B. Nonadherence to asthma treatment: getting unstuck. J Allergy Clin Immunol Pract 2016;4:849–51.

10. Morton RW, Everard ML, Elphick HE. Adherence in childhood asthma: the elephant in the room. Arch Dis Child 2014;99:949–53.

11. Morawska A, Stelzer J, Burgess S. Parenting asthmatic children: identification of parenting challenges. J Asthma 2008;45:465–72.

12. Walders N, Kopel SJ, Koinis-Mitchell D, et al. Patterns of quick-relief and long-term controller medication use in pediatric asthma. J Pediatr 2005;146:177–82.

13. Otsuki-Clutter M, Sutter M, Ewig J. Promoting adherence to inhaled corticosteroid therapy in patients with asthma. J Clin Outcomes Manage 2011;18:177–82.

14. Miles C, Arden-Close E, Thomas M, et al. Barriers and facilitators of effective self-management in asthma: systematic review and thematic synthesis of patient and healthcare professional views. NPJ Prim Care Respir Med 2017;27:57.

15. Modi AC, Pai AL, Hommel KA, et al. Pediatric self-management: a framework for research, practice, and policy. Pediatrics 2012;129:e473–85.

16. Sonney J, Insel KC. Exploring the intersection of executive function and medication adherence in school-age children with asthma. J Asthma 2018;7:1–22.

17. Pai AL, McGrady M. Systematic review and meta-analysis of psychological interventions to promote adherence in children, adolescents, and young adults with chronic illness. J Pediatr Psychol 2014;39:918–31.

18. Kahana S, Drotar D, Frazier T. Meta-analysis of psychological interventions to promote adherence to treatment in pediatric chronic health conditions. J Pediatr Psychol 2008;33:590–611.

19. Modi AC, Quittner AL. Barriers to treatment adherence for children with cystic fibrosis and asthma: what gets in the way? J Pediatr Psychol 2006;31:846–58.

20. Burgess SW, Sly PD, Morasawka A, et al. Assessing adherence and factors associated with adherence in young children with asthma. Respirology 2008;13: 559–63.

21. Calam R, Gregg L, Goodman R. Psychological adjustment and asthma in children and adolescents: the UK nationwide mental health survey. Psychosom Med 2005;67:105–10.

22. Calam R, Gregg L, Simpson BM, et al. Childhood asthma, behavior problems, and family functioning. J Allergy Clin Immunol 2003;112:499–504.

23. Koinis-Mitchell D, McQuaid EL, Seifer R, et al. Symptom perception in children with asthma: cognitive and psychological factors. Health Psychol 2009;28: 226–37.

24. Chen E, Hermann C, Rodgers D, et al. Symptom perception in childhood asthma: the role of anxiety and asthma severity. Health Psychol 2006;25:389–95.

25. Berg CJ, Rapoff MA, Synder CR, et al. The relationship of children's hope to pediatric asthma treatment adherence. J Posit Psychol 2007;2:176–84.

26. Englund A-CD, Rydstrom I, Norberg A. Being the parent of a child with asthma. Pediatr Nurs 2001;27:365–75.

27. Pappalardo AA, Karavolos K, Martin MA. What really happens in the home: The medication environment of urban, minority youth. J Allergy Clin Immunol Pract 2016;5:764–70.

28. Mirsadraee R, Gharagozlou M, Movahedi M, et al. Evaluation of factors contributed in nonadherence to medication therapy in children asthma. Iran J Allergy Asthma Immunol 2012;11:23–7.

29. Friend M, Morrison A. Interventions to improve asthma management of the school-age child. Clin Pediatr (Phila) 2015;54:534–42.

30. Zedan M, Regal MEE, Osman EA, et al. Steroid phobia among parents of asthmatic children: myths and truth. Iran J Allergy Asthma Immunol 2010;9:163–8.

31. Bender B. Risk taking, depression, adherence, and symptom control in adolescents and young adults with asthma. Am J Respir Crit Care Med 2006;173:953–7.

32. Katon W, Lozano P, Russo J, et al. The prevalence of DSM-IV anxiety and depressive disorders in youth with asthma compared with controls. J Adolesc Health 2007;41:455–63.

33. McQuaid EL, Kopel SJ, Nassau JH. Behavioral adjustment in children with asthma: a meta-analysis. J Dev Behav Pediatr 2001;22:430–9.

34. Haltermann JS, Yoos HL, Conn KM, et al. The impact of childhood asthma on parental quality of life. J Asthma 2004;41:645–53.

35. Feldman JM, Steinberg D, Kutner H, et al. Perception of pulmonary function and asthma control: the differential role of child versus caregiver anxiety and depression. J Pediatr Psychol 2013;38:1091–100.

36. Lim JH, Wood BL, Miller BD, et al. Effects of paternal and maternal depressive symptoms on child internalizing symptoms and asthma disease activity: mediation by interparental negativity and parenting. J Fam Psychol 2011;35:137–46.

37. Di Matteo MR, Lepper HS, Croghan TW. Depression is a risk factor for noncompliance with medical treatment: meta-analysis of the effects of anxiety and depression on patient adherence. Arch Intern Med 2000;160:2101–7.

38. Booster G, Oland A, Bender B. Psychosocial factors in severe pediatric asthma. Immunol Allergy Clin North Am 2016;36:449–60.

39. Wade SL. Psychosocial components of asthma management in children. Dis Manag Health Outcome 2000;8:17–27.

40. Wamboldt FS, Wamboldt MZ, Gavin LA, et al. Parental criticism and treatment outcome in adolescents hospitalized for severe, chronic asthma. J Psychosom Res 1995;39:995–1005.
41. Kaugars AS, Klinnert MD, Bender BG. Family influences on pediatric asthma. J Pediatr Psychol 2004;29:475–91.
42. Warman K, Silver EJ, Wood PR. Asthma risk factor assessment: what are the needs of inner city families? Ann Allergy Asthma Immunol 2006;97(Suppl):S11–5.
43. Lucas SR, Platts-Mills TA. Physical activity and exercise in asthma: relevance to etiology and treatment. J Allergy Clin Immunol 2005;115:928–34.
44. Halterman JS, Auinger P, Conn KM, et al. Inadequate therapy and poor symptom control among children with asthma: Findings from a multistate sample. Ambul Pediatr 2007;7:153–9.
45. Celano MP, Linzer JF, Demi A, et al. Treatment adherence among low-income, African American children with persistent asthma. J Asthma 2010;47:317–22.
46. Basch CE. Asthma and the achievement gap among urban minority youth. J Sch Health 2011;81:606–13.
47. Peterson-Sweeney K, McMullen A, Yoos HL, et al. Parental perceptions of their children's asthma: management and medication use. J Pediatr Health Care 2003;17:118–25.
48. Duncan CL, Walker HA, Brabson L, et al. Developing pictorial asthma action plans to promote self-management and health in rural youth with asthma: a qualitative study. J Asthma 2018;55(8):915–23.
49. Valet RS, Perry TT, Hartert TV. Rural health disparities in asthma care and outcomes. J Allergy Clin Immunol 2009;123:1220–5.
50. Agency for Healthcare Research and Quality. 2012 national healthcare disparities report. 2013. Available at: http://www.ahrq.gov/research/findings/nhqrdr/nhdr12/2012nhdr.pdf. Accessed April 1, 2017.
51. Sandel M, Wright RJ. When home is where the stress is: expanding the dimensions of housing that influence asthma morbidity. Arch Dis Child 2006;91:942–8.
52. Sheehan WJ, Philatanakul W. Difficult-to-control asthma: epidemiology and its link with environmental factors. Curr Opin Allergy Clin Immunol 2015;15:397–401.
53. Adler NE, Conner Snibbe A. The role of psychosocial processes in explaining the gradient between socioeconomic status and health. Curr Dir Psychol Sci 2003;12:119–23.
54. Wright RJ. Health effects of socially toxic neighborhoods; the violence and urban asthma paradigm. Clin Chest Med 2006;27:413–21.
55. Chen E, Fisher E, Bacharier LB, et al. Socioeconomic status, stress, and immune markers in adolescents with asthma. Psychosom Med 2003;65:984–92.
56. Marin TJ, Chen E, Munch JA, et al. Double-exposure to acute stress and chronic family stress is associated with immune changes in children with asthma. Psychosom Med 2009;71:378–84.
57. Otsuki M, Eakin MN, Rand CS, et al. Adherence feedback to improve asthma outcomes among inner-city children: a randomized trial. Pediatrics 2009;124:1513–21.
58. Morton RW, Elphick HE, Rigby AS, et al. STAAR: a randomized controlled trial of electronic adherence monitoring with reminder alarms and feedback to improve clinical outcomes for children with asthma. Thorax 2017;72:347–54.
59. Apter AJ, Morales KH, Han X, et al. A patient advocate to facilitate access and improve communication, care, and outcomes in adults with moderate or severe asthma: rationale, design, and methods of a randomized controlled trial. Contemp Clin Trials 2017;56:34–45.

60. Fox P, Porter PG, Lob SH, et al. Improving asthma-related health outcomes among low-income, multiethnic, school-aged children: Results of a demonstration project that combined continuous quality improvement and community health worker strategies. Pediatrics 2007;120:e902–11.
61. Andreae SJ, Andreae LJ, Cherrington AL, et al. Development of a community health worker-delivered cognitive behavioral training intervention for individuals with diabetes and chronic pain. Fam Community Health 2018;41:178–84.
62. Normansell R, Kew KM, Stovold E. Interventions to improve adherence to inhaled steroids for asthma (review). Cochrane Database Syst Rev 2017;(4):CD012226.
63. Chuenjit W, Engchuan V, Yuenyongviwat A, et al. Achieving good adherence to inhaled corticosteroids after weighing canisters of asthmatic children. F1000Res 2017;6:266.
64. Spaulding SA, Devine KA, Duncan CL, et al. Electronic monitoring and feedback to improve adherence in pediatric asthma. J Pediatr Psychol 2012;37:64–74.
65. Burgess SW, Sly PD, Devadason SG. Providing feedback on adherence increases use of preventative medication by asthmatic children. J Asthma 2010; 47:198–201.
66. Wiecha JM, Adams WG, Rybin D, et al. Evaluation of a web-based asthma self-management system: a randomized controlled pilot trial. BMC Pulm Med 2015;15–7. https://doi.org/10.1186/s12890-015-0007-1.
67. Elias P, Rajan NO, McArthur K, et al. InSpire to promote lung assessment in youth: Evolving the self-management paradigms of young people with asthma. Med 2.0 2013;2:e1.
68. Roter DL, Hall JA, Merisca R, et al. Effectiveness of interventions to improve patient compliance: a meta-analysis. Med Care 1998;36:1138–61.
69. Burkhart PV, Rayens MK, Oakley MG, et al. Testing and intervention to promote children's adherence to asthma self-management. J Nurs Scholarsh 2007;39: 133–40.
70. Da Costa IG, Rapoff MA, Lemanek K, et al. Improving adherence to medication regimens for children with asthma and its effect on clinical outcome. J Appl Behav Anal 1997;30:687–91.
71. Rohan JM, Drotar D, Perry AR, et al. Training health care providers to conduct adherence promotion in pediatric settings: an example with pediatric asthma. Clin Pract Ped Psychol 2013;1:314–25.
72. Morawska A, Mitchell AE, Burgess S, et al. Effects of triple P parenting intervention on child health outcomes for childhood asthma and eczema: randomized controlled trial. Behav Res Ther 2016;83:35–44.
73. Halterman JS, Fagnano M, Tajon RS, et al. Effect of the school-based telemedicine enhanced asthma management (SB-TEAM) program on asthma morbidity: a randomized clinical trial. JAMA Pediatr 2018;173:e174938.
74. Trivedi M, Patel J, Lessard D, et al. School nurse asthma program reduces healthcare utilization in children with persistent asthma. J Asthma 2017;5:1–7.
75. Rapoff M. Adherence to pediatric medical regimens. New York: Springer; 2010.
76. Israel B, Coombe C, Cheezum R, et al. Community-based participatory research: a capacity-building approach for policy advocacy aimed at eliminating health disparities. Am J Public Health 2010;100:2094–102.
77. Kelleher C, Riley-Tillman TC, Power TJ. An initial comparison of collaborative and expert driven consultation on treatment integrity. J Educ Psychol Consult 2008; 18:294–324.

Severe Asthma in Childhood

Angela Marko, DO[a], Kristie R. Ross, MD, MS[b],*

KEYWORDS

- Severe asthma • Children • Phenotype • Management

KEY POINTS

- Severe asthma in childhood is a heterogeneous condition, but is broadly defined as asthma that requires a high level of therapy to achieve control.
- Asthma phenotypes and endotypes are important to stratify clinical features, underlying pathophysiological mechanisms, and treatment responses and are essential to guide future therapeutic development.
- Management of a child with severe asthma requires a detailed multidisciplinary assessment.

INTRODUCTION

Childhood asthma, characterized by airway inflammation, hyperresponsiveness, and variable airflow obstruction, affects 8.4% of all children younger than 18 years in the United States.[1,2] Although many children with asthma respond well to standard therapies, such as short-acting bronchodilators and daily inhaled corticosteroids (ICSs), a substantial minority do not.[3] Severe asthma in childhood is a heterogeneous condition, but is broadly defined as asthma that requires a high level of therapy to achieve control.[4,5] The prevalence of severe asthma in children is estimated to be approximately 5% to 10% of the total asthma population.[4] However, the burden on these children and the health care system is quite high, with the annual cost of caring for these children estimated to be more than half of all asthma-related health care expenditures, primarily due to much higher resource utilization.[6]

The definition of severe asthma proposed in the American Thoracic Society (ATS) and European Respiratory Society (ERS) guideline document does not differ among

Dr K.R. Ross reports research grants to her institution from the National Institutes of Health and the Ohio Department of Jobs and Family Services relevant to the current work, nonfinancial support from TEVA, Glaxo Smith Kline, Boehringer Ingelheim, and Astra Zeneca for the conduct of clinical studies related to the current work, and grants for the conduct of clinical trials from Jazz not related to the current work. Dr A. Marko has no conflicts to disclose.
[a] Division of Pediatric Pulmonology, University Hospitals Rainbow Babies and Children's Hospital, 11100 Euclid Avenue, Cleveland, OH 44106, USA; [b] Division of Pediatric Pulmonology, University Hospitals Rainbow Babies and Children's Hospital, Case Western Reserve University School of Medicine, 11100 Euclid Avenue, Cleveland, OH 44106, USA
* Corresponding author.
E-mail address: Kristie.ross@uhhospitals.org

Immunol Allergy Clin N Am 39 (2019) 243–257
https://doi.org/10.1016/j.iac.2018.12.007
0889-8561/19/© 2018 Elsevier Inc. All rights reserved.

immunology.theclinics.com

children, adolescents, and adults, apart from age-specific thresholds of ICS dose that meet the designation of high-dose treatment.[4] Children and adolescents who either remain uncontrolled when treated with high-dose ICS plus a second controller, systemic corticosteroids for more than 50% of the year, or a biologic therapy are defined as having severe asthma. Lack of control is defined broadly; a patient is considered to be uncontrolled if he or she has at least 1 of the following:

1. A high symptom burden using the Asthma Control Questionnaire or the Asthma Control Test
2. Two or more exacerbations requiring oral corticosteroids in the previous year
3. One or more hospitalization, intensive care unit stay, or episode requiring mechanical ventilation in the past year
4. Airflow limitation (reduced forced expiratory volume in 1 second [FEV_1]/forced vital capacity (FVC) ratio with FEV_1 <80% predicted) following a bronchodilator hold

Children who are controlled while on high-level therapies but lose control with attempts at tapering also meet criteria for severe asthma.

Unlike other chronic conditions that can be staged or graded using objective testing, the definition of severe asthma is based on a determination that the disease is refractory to treatment. This requires that medications are prescribed and taken correctly, comorbid conditions that can influence response to therapy have been evaluated and managed, and that alternative diagnoses that may mimic asthma but would not respond to therapy have been considered. From a practical standpoint, these steps are best accomplished by specialist evaluation and management before making the diagnosis of severe asthma, as suggested in the ATS/ERS guidelines.[4] Approximately half of children referred for severe asthma have an alternative or comorbid diagnosis and/or modifiable factors that when addressed reduce asthma severity.[7]

Much of the work showing the importance of a multistaged and interdisciplinary approach to the child with difficult asthma has been done in the context of universal access to health care.[8,9] In the United States, where a significant proportion of asthma care for some populations is delivered in the emergency room setting,[10] the distinction between asthma that is difficult to treat due to comorbid and/or modifiable factors and severe treatment refractory asthma is important at the population health level, but may be challenging to address at the individual patient level.

It is also worth highlighting that many of the children who die from an asthma exacerbation do not necessarily meet the guideline definition of severe asthma, but few would argue that fatal and near fatal asthma represent a severe form of the disease. Children who die from acute asthma are likely a heterogeneous population, ranging from children who have been undertreated because of poor access to care or underrecognition of symptoms, children with high exposures to irritants and/or allergens, children who have severe infections, and children with inherent treatment-refractory severe asthma. The strongest risk factor for a severe exacerbation is a past severe exacerbation,[11,12] suggesting exacerbation-prone asthma may be a distinct phenotype.[13]

EPIDEMIOLOGY

Although there is heterogeneity in severe childhood asthma, more than two-thirds of children with asthma have allergic sensitization.[14] Early sensitization to foods and aeroallergens is an important determinant of persistent asthma by school age.[15,16] Several studies have shown that atopy is increased in children with severe asthma compared with mild asthma,[17] in contrast to adults in which the opposite pattern is seen. Allergic sensitization also plays an important role in asthma exacerbations, best exemplified by the ability of anti-immunoglobulin (Ig)E to reduce the burst of ex-acerbations seen in children in early fall.[18]

In addition to atopy, male sex,[19] maternal or paternal history of asthma,[20] preterm birth,[21] overweight/obesity,[22] minority race,[23] and socioeconomic and geographic factors[24,25] are all well-established risk factors for childhood asthma. There are con-flicting reports in the literature with respect to these risk factors and asthma severity and response to treatment, likely due to important interactions with genetic back-ground. For example, in the Severe Asthma Research Program (SARP) III cohort, chil-dren with severe and nonsevere asthma were similar in terms of race, sex, and body mass index,[14] whereas earlier pediatric SARP cohorts found nonwhite children were more likely to be categorized as severe.[26] Racial and economic disparities and other social determinants of health are important contributors to health care utilization and asthma-related morbidity in the United States[25,27–31]; whether there are intrinsic differ-ences in asthma severity due to these factors has yet to be determined. However, the impact of adverse life experiences and other prenatal and perinatal exposures more common in poor and minority children on lung development and asthma suggest that there may be lasting biological effects.[32–35]

PATHOPHYSIOLOGY

Asthma is characterized by airway hyperreactivity, obstruction, and inflammation. Hallmarks of pulmonary physiology in severe asthma include structural abnormalities that affect airway mechanics, including airflow, airway resistance, air trapping, lung elastic recoil, and bronchial hyperresponsiveness.[4] Many adults with severe asthma are characterized by marked airway obstruction that may be "fixed" (ie, not fully reversible with bronchodilators), particularly in those with early-onset atopic dis-ease.[34] Children in the SARP, who were largely atopic and by definition had childhood-onset disease, had evidence for some airway obstruction but it was much less severe than that seen in adults.[5] Bronchodilator responsiveness was also largely preserved even in children with other features of severe asthma,[5] suggesting the development of fixed airway obstruction generally occurs after childhood. Children in the more severe phenotypes in the SARP were more likely to have bronchial hyper-responsiveness and air trapping.[5,6] Whether children with severe disease and early airway obstruction will go on to become adults with moderate to severe fixed airway obstruction is an open question, although there are studies to suggest this progression can occur.[26,36] Decreased lung recoil is considered an important determinant in airflow limitation, as this contributes to airway narrowing.[37] The exact mechanism for this is unknown, but remodeling of the airway outer wall and an increased propor-tion of abnormal alveolar attachments has been reported in patients with fatal asthma.[38] Abnormalities in structural airway cells also contribute to abnormal inflam-mation and airway mechanics. Early thickening of the reticular basement membrane (RBM) has been described in children with severe asthma.[39] Other components of airway remodeling observed in children with severe asthma include larger smooth muscle area, increased MLCK expression (protein involved in smooth muscle contrac-tion), shorter distance between smooth muscle and RBM, and increased density of the vascular network.[40] Patients with severe asthma also have been observed to have increased transforming growth factor (TGF)-β as well as alterations in collagen depo-sition.[40,41] It remains unclear if there is a direct link between airway remodeling and airway inflammation, especially in children with severe disease.[39,40]

Airway inflammation is a consistent feature of asthma. The dominant cell type found in the airways can be used to characterize airway inflammation, and in adults with severe asthma, the distinction between eosinophilic, neutrophilic, and paucigranulo-cytic disease may inform treatment response.[41] Although some studies have shown associations between the dominant cell type in bronchoalveolar lavage fluid and endo-bronchial biopsies in children and a particular phenotype of severe asthma,[42,43] others have not.[42,44] Molecular phenotypes have also been difficult to define in severe child-hood asthma.[44,45] The lack of stability of cellular inflammation in children[46] and the challenges in assessing it limit the clinical use.[42,43,45,47,48]

With evidence mounting that an imbalance between Th1 and Th2 adaptive immunity is not sufficient to explain the development of childhood asthma or the severe presen-tation of childhood asthma, and the recognition of the important role viral infections play in the inception of childhood asthma and during exacerbations, there is intense study of immune dysregulation in asthma outside the classic Th2 paradigm. Areas of interest that may inform the development of new therapies to meet this high unmet need include airway macrophage dysfunction,[44] oxidative stress,[49,50] profibrotic signaling including TGF-β1 expression and activation,[50] nonallergic inflammation including tumor necrosis factor-α,[46] impaired or altered response to viral infec-tions,[44,49,51] and alterations in the microbiome.[50]

CLINICAL FEATURES

Taken as a whole, children with severe asthma are generally atopic with at least some ev-idence for eosinophilic airway inflammation.[5,52] Despite these generally shared features, other characteristics of severe childhood asthma are heterogeneous, with mismatch be-tween domains of impairment and risk.[53] The clinical characteristics, or phenotypes, of severe asthma have been described using both hypothesis-driven and unsupervised ap-proaches.[4,52,54–61] Cluster analysis of children with severe and nonsevere asthma enrolled in the cross-sectional SARP showed children aggregated into 1 of 4 clusters:

1. Early-onset atopic with normal lung function
2. Early-onset atopic with mild airflow limitation
3. Early-onset with advanced airflow limitation
4. Later-onset with normal lung function[26]

Clusters 3 and 4 had high proportions of children with severe asthma using ATS-ERS criteria. Health care utilization was high in all clusters, but children in clusters 3 and 4 had more unscheduled visits for acute symptoms and more frequent courses of sys-temic corticosteroids. Separate analysis of children enrolled in the longitudinal Child-hood Asthma Management Program (CAMP) found 5 clusters of childhood asthma differentiated by atopic burden, degree of airway obstruction, and history of exacerba-tions.[52] Although there was 1 cluster characterized as "low" atopy, more than 75% of children in this cluster had positive skin tests. The long-term follow-up data available in CAMP allowed researchers to show the stability of cluster assignment over time, which has not yet been done with the SARP clusters. Children assigned to clusters 4 and 5 (the most severe clusters) had the highest risk for exacerbations during prospective follow-up. Investigators also showed some evidence that phenotype predicted treat-ment response in the randomized clinical trial portion of CAMP, in which children were randomized to daily budesonide, nedocromil, or placebo. Children in the less se-vere clusters 1 to 3 responded best to budesonide; however, children in cluster 4 responded better to nedocromil than either budesonide or placebo, and children in cluster 5 had equal response to budesonide, nedocromil, and placebo.[52] Others have shown that assigning phenotype using the SARP cluster definitions may also help predict response to therapy in clinical trials, with children assigned to clusters 3 and 4 having more limited response to treatments across several studies in the National Heart Lung and Blood Institute's (NHLBI) Childhood Asthma Research (CARE) Network.[55] Work is under way now to extend phenotype analyses to include underlying biological mechanisms, known as endotypes, that may help better target therapies.[44,52,56–64] The NHLBI recently funded the Precision Interventions for Severe and/ or Exacerbation Prone Asthma (PreclSE) Network to study targeted treatments in adults and adolescents with severe asthma using these concepts.

Differential Diagnosis and Diagnosis Confirmation

Evaluating severe asthma in children requires a comprehensive approach, beginning establishing that asthma is the most likely cause of symptoms using a comprehensive history, physical examination, and noninvasive testing. Confirming the presence of classic triggers (viral infections, play/exercise, allergens, irritants), typical symptom patterns and response (worse at night, responsive to bronchodilators and previous trials of ICS or other asthma controller medications), and lack of symptoms and signs suggesting disease other than asthma (eg, productive cough, breathlessness without cough, recurrent sinopulmonary or other infections, failure to thrive, clubbing) are important steps. Assessments of the home and school environment, family history, and for comorbid conditions that may modify response to treatment are also important early steps. Multiple studies have shown high rates of alternative diagnoses in children evaluated using comprehensive approaches[57,58]; therefore, it is important that clinicians maintain a high index of suspicion for conditions that may masquerade as severe asthma (**Box 1**). Assessment of adherence to prescribed medications and the self-management plan include regular use of controller medications, adequate device

---

Box 1
Conditions that may mimic asthma

Tracheomalacia/bronchomalacia

Oropharyngeal dysfunction and aspiration

Retained foreign body

Vocal cord dysfunction or dysfunctional breathing

Extrinsic airway compression

Congenital airway anomaly

Airway masses/tumors

Immune deficiency

Primary ciliary dyskinesia

Childhood diffuse lung disease

Suppurative lung disease (non–cystic fibrosis bronchiectasis, chronic bacterial bronchitis)

Anxiety/panic disorder

Chronic lung disease of prematurity

Pulmonary vascular disease

Pulmonary eosinophilic syndrome

Allergic bronchopulmonary aspergillosis

Hypersensitivity pneumonitis

Obliterative bronchiolitis

technique, avoidance of triggers when possible, and the ability to problem solve during loss of asthma control and exacerbations are also key steps.[9,58,59]

Spirometry is used to confirm reversible airflow limitation. Testing should include both inspiratory and expiratory loops before and after bronchodilator therapy to assess for presence of reversibility and to help evaluate for upper airway obstruction (eg, vocal cord dysfunction). Ideally, this should be done in the absence of any recent short-acting or long-acting bronchodilators to best assess responsiveness.[4,59] Spirometry is ideally done before initiation of controller therapies, but as children are frequently not referred for testing before initiation of ICS, the clinical context should be considered in interpretation. Children with severe asthma may have normal lung function and may not show reversibility to bronchodilators on spirometry when well.[5,26,60] Bacharier and colleagues[52] reported that FEV_1% predicted did not differ with asthma severity; however, FEV_1/FVC decreased as asthma severity increased. There are also age-related diagnostic challenges in children younger than 6 years. With proper coaching and practice, pulmonary function tests may be possible in young children, although limited reference data exist for this age group.[61] Given the very high prevalence of atopy in children with severe asthma, testing for allergic sensitization with either skin prick testing or allergen-specific IgE should be done.[54,62] **Fig. 1** presents a framework for the consideration of additional testing when clinically indicated in challenging or atypical cases.[4,59]

MANAGEMENT

International guidelines recommend a stepwise approach to the management of asthma in children and adults.[54,62] As discussed previously and described in these guidelines, assessment of adherence to the current treatment plan and for modifiable

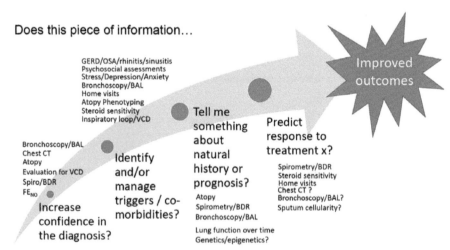

Fig. 1. Framework for the diagnostic and monitoring approach to the child with severe asthma. Evaluation should be directed based on the child's specific symptoms and signs, with consideration of the potential risks. Advanced diagnostic testing may be helpful in establishing the diagnosis of asthma or an alternative diagnosis, identifying modifiable factors that may impact response to therapy, provide prognostic information, or predict response to specific treatments. BAL, bronchoalveolar lavage; BDR, bronchodilator reversibility; CT, computed tomography; FE_{NO}, fractional exhaled nitric oxide; GERD, gastroesophageal disease; OSA, obstructive sleep apnea; VCD, vocal cord dysfunction.

factors limiting the effectiveness of treatment is recommended before escalation of therapy.[8,62,63] Work in the United Kingdom and by others makes a distinction between difficult-to-treat asthma in which modifiable factors such as adherence, environmental conditions, and comorbid conditions (shown in **Fig. 2**) impact response, and asthma that is intrinsically refractory to currently available therapies. Much of this work has been done in the setting of universal access to care.[8,59,64] In environments in which the ability to modify social determinants of health is limited by system financial issues, distinguishing between difficult-to-treat and therapy-resistant asthma is important but may be challenging. Advocacy efforts to impact health policy are critical in this regard. A detailed discussion on adherence monitoring and management, the role of the environment, and the approach to assessment and management of comorbidities (see **Fig. 2**) (see Carolyn Kercsmar and Cassie Shipp article's, "Management/ Comorbidities of School-Aged Children with Asthma," can be found elsewhere in this issue). The role of each of these steps is particularly important in children with severe asthma, given the potential for adverse effects as therapies are escalated.

After assessment as outlined previously, treatment with high-dose ICS plus a long-acting beta-agonist, leukotriene modifier, theophylline, biologic therapies, and/or prolonged use of oral corticosteroids are used in children with severe asthma to achieve control.[4,54,65] Treatment responses vary substantially, and the approach to personalized therapies is covered in detail in the article by Guilbert and Pajor, elsewhere in this issue. Assessment of steroid responsiveness and partnering with the child and family to understand the treatment goals they identify as most important may be helpful. Bossley and colleagues[66] demonstrated that complete response to systemic steroids was rare, with 72% determined to be partial responders and 15% nonresponders, supporting the concept of disease heterogeneity of the disease and the importance of determining treatment response across domains that include symptoms, lung function, exacerbations, and airway inflammation.

In cases in which there is minimal-to-no steroid response or concerns for adverse effects from steroid use, the use of anticholinergics and biological agents should be

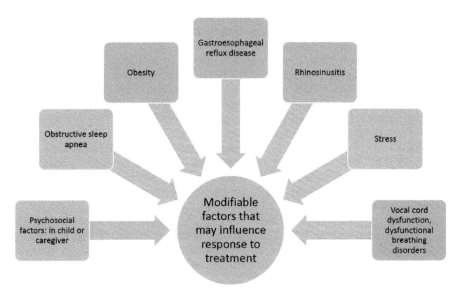

Fig. 2. Comorbid conditions that may influence response therapy and, when addressed, may distinguish difficult-to-treat asthma from asthma that is intrinsically refractive to therapies.

considered.[4,59,67] Tiotropium is a long-acting anticholinergic used as an add-on therapy in moderate-to-severe asthma that has been approved for use in those 6 years and older. A recent systematic review demonstrated that once-daily tiotropium was efficacious and well tolerated as an add-on medication in school-aged children with symptomatic asthma.[67] In addition to this, new biological agents provide a more phenotype/endotype-directed strategy for those with severe asthma.

There are currently 3 monoclonal antibodies approved for children and adolescents. Omalizumab is a monoclonal antibody to IgE, is approved for children and adolescents ≥6 years old with allergic sensitization, and has the longest track record for efficacy and safety in children with multiple clinical trials and real-world use studies showing reduced exacerbations and hospitalizations, improved lung function, a steroid-sparing effect, and fewer adverse events than placebo other than injection site reactions.[53,68] Omalizumab also reduces the fall exacerbation phenomenon in allergic children with asthma, with evidence for specific effects against rhinovirus infection.[18,69,70] Although studies of omalizumab have included those with moderate and severe asthma, the cost and burden of treatment (injections given every 2–4 weeks under medical supervision due to concerns about anaphylaxis) has generally limited its use to those with more severe disease.

Another class of biologics includes mepolizumab and benralizumab, which target either interleukin (IL)-5 ligand or receptor, respectively, are recommended as an adjunct in those with persistent eosinophilic inflammation. Mepolizumab is a monoclonal antibody against IL-5, which disrupts eosinophil maturation resulting in reduction of eosinophils in sputum and blood. It is currently approved for children ≥12 years old with blood eosinophils ≥150 cells per µL, and is dosed every 4 weeks. Several studies have demonstrated that mepolizumab significantly reduces the number of asthma exacerbations[71] and has significant glucocorticoid-sparing effects in patients with severe eosinophilic asthma compared with placebo.[72] In addition, another study demonstrated that treatment with either intravenous or subcutaneous doses was effective at reducing exacerbations and improving quality of life.[73]

Similarly, benralizumab is an anti-eosinophilic monoclonal antibody; however, its target is IL-5 receptor α. In contrast to other therapies that target IL-5 directly and only reduce eosinophils, benralizumab targets the receptor, thus resulting in rapid eosinophilic depletion.[74] It is currently approved for children ≥12 years old with severe or uncontrolled asthma with eosinophilia. Clinical trials have demonstrated that benralizumab was well tolerated, as seen by low discontinuation rate and had few drug-related adverse events.[75] Additional potential advantages of benralizumab include its direct action to deplete blood eosinophils compared with the indirect action of those medicines that target the IL-5 ligand (mepolizumab and reslizumab), as well as every 8-week dosing interval to help lower disease burden and health care costs compared with other biologics.[74] Findings from 2 studies showed benralizumab resulted in substantial improvements in asthma exacerbations, lung function, and symptom control when used as add-on therapy for patients with severe, uncontrolled asthma with elevated baseline blood eosinophils.

Dupilumab, an monoclonal antibody to the alpha subunit of the IL-4 receptor, resulting in reduction in IL-4 and IL-13, is currently under review at the Food and Drug Administration for the treatment of moderate to severe asthma in patients ≥12 years old based on clinical trials showing steroid-sparing effects,[76] reduced exacerbations, and improved lung function.[77] Data in adolescents for mepolizumab, benralizumab, and dupilumab are quite limited, with a small number of adolescents included in the major clinical trials for each.

PROGNOSIS

The goals of treatment of severe childhood asthma include symptom and exacerbation management, but as pediatricians we are also concerned with prevention of progression of asthma into adulthood. Cross-sectional data and data from the longitudinal SARP III cohort suggest that many children with severe asthma experience at least a transient improvement in asthma severity during adolescence and early adulthood.[78–80] However, this improvement does not include lung function deficits, and children with a range of asthma severity and treatment may develop irreversible obstruction or chronic obstructive pulmonary disease (COPD).[81,82] In a landmark longitudinal analysis of children with mild to moderate asthma enrolled in the CAMP study, only 25% had normal lung function patterns in early adulthood, with the remaining participants showing either reduced growth, early decline, or both.[81] More than 1 in 10 met criteria for COPD in their early 20s. Impaired lung function at enrollment and male sex were the strongest predictors for abnormal lung function in early adulthood. These findings suggest that even mild to moderate asthma in early life impacts lifelong health.[81] Although the longitudinal analysis of lung function in the CAMP study included only those with mild-to-moderate asthma, some studies have shown the risk for COPD is higher in children with more severe disease.[83,84] Data from the SARP suggests irreversible obstruction is less common in children than in adults,[85] and additional study of effective strategies to prevent lung function decline is an important area of unmet need.[86]

ADVOCACY

Severe asthma is tightly linked with socioeconomic status and minority race and ethnicity in the United States. Markers of asthma severity, including emergency room use, hospitalizations, and deaths due to asthma are all substantially higher in poor and minority populations than their more affluent white peers.[87,88] Implementation of guidelines-based care with good adherence to standard therapies results in improved asthma control even in high-risk populations,[89] although high rates of difficult-to-control asthma may persist even in the setting of a clinical trial.[90] The underlying causes of asthma disparities are complex,[25] but include environmental exposures at home and in schools (allergens, indoor and outdoor air pollution),[91] neighborhood level factors,[92] access to care and treatment,[93,94] caretaker stress and mental health,[95] and financial and social hardships.[96] Although interventions that address the social determinants of health relevant to asthma reduce morbidity,[97–100] sustaining these programs outside the context of clinical research is challenging and requires health care providers and institutions to form partnerships with legal professionals, community-based programs, insurance programs, and legislators.[101–104] Given the high cost of biological therapies for asthma, we suggest these types of collaborations and advocacy on behalf of our patients with severe asthma are a component of personalized medicine that should not be overlooked.

SUMMARY

Children with severe asthma require a detailed medical workup, careful consideration of alternative diagnoses, assessment of adherence to medications and self-management plans, and evaluation of comorbid conditions. This multidisciplinary approach is critical to optimize care in this high-risk severe asthma population. Further research and validation of phenotype/endotype clusters in more longitudinal studies are an important next step. These efforts are essential to develop frameworks to classify severe asthma, personalize therapy, and develop new strategies that address unmet needs. The role of social determinants of health and advocacy for health policies that address modifiable factors is a critical part of the care of children with severe asthma.

REFERENCES

1. Lemanske RF, Busse WW. Asthma: clinical expression and molecular mechanisms. J Allergy Clin Immunol 2010;125(2):S95–102.
2. Centers for Disease Control and Prevention. CDC - asthma - Table 4-1 current asthma prevalence percents by age. Atlanta (GA): NHIS; 2015. Available at: https://www.cdc.gov/asthma/nhis/2015/table4-1.htm. Accessed May 5, 2018.
3. Childhood Asthma Management Program Research Group, Szefler S, Weiss S, Tonascia J, et al. Long-term effects of budesonide or nedocromil in children with asthma. N Engl J Med 2000;343(15):1054–63.
4. Chung KF, Wenzel SE, Brozek JL, et al. International ERS/ATS guidelines on definition, evaluation and treatment of severe asthma. Eur Respir J 2014; 43(2):343–73.
5. Fitzpatrick AM, Gaston BM, Erzurum SC, et al, National Institutes of Health/National Heart, Lung, and Blood Institute Severe Asthma Research Program. Features of severe asthma in school-age children: atopy and increased exhaled nitric oxide. J Allergy Clin Immunol 2006;118(6):1218–25.
6. Haselkorn T, Fish JE, Zeiger RS, et al. Consistently very poorly controlled asthma, as defined by the impairment domain of the Expert Panel Report 3 guidelines, increases risk for future severe asthma exacerbations in The Epidemiology and Natural History of Asthma: Outcomes and Treatment Regimens (TENOR) study. J Allergy Clin Immunol 2009;124(5):895–902.e1-4.
7. Bossley CJ, Saglani S, Kavanagh C, et al. Corticosteroid responsiveness and clinical characteristics in childhood difficult asthma. Eur Respir J 2009;34(5): 1052–9.
8. Bush A, Fleming L, Saglani S. Severe asthma in children. Respirology 2017; 22(5):886–97.
9. Jochmann A, Artusio L, Jamalzadeh A, et al. Electronic monitoring of adherence to inhaled corticosteroids: an essential tool in identifying severe asthma in children. Eur Respir J 2017;50(6):1700910.
10. Stingone JA, Claudio L. Disparities in the use of urgent health care services among asthmatic children. Ann Allergy Asthma Immunol 2006;97(2):244–50.
11. Alvarez G, Schulzer M, Jung D, et al. A systematic review of risk factors associated with near-fatal and fatal asthma. Can Respir J 2005;12(5):265–70.
12. Haselkorn T, Zeiger RS, Chipps BE, et al. Recent asthma exacerbations predict future exacerbations in children with severe or difficult-to-treat asthma. J Allergy Clin Immunol 2009;124(5):921–7.
13. Denlinger LC, Phillips BR, Ramratnam S, et al. Inflammatory and comorbid features of patients with severe asthma and frequent exacerbations. Am J Respir Crit Care Med 2017;195(3):302–13.
14. Teague WG, Phillips BR, Fahy JV, et al. Baseline features of the Severe Asthma Research Program (SARP III) cohort: differences with age. J Allergy Clin Immunol Pract 2018;6(2):545–54.e4.
15. Heymann PW, Carper HT, Murphy DD, et al. Viral infections in relation to age, atopy, and season of admission among children hospitalized for wheezing. J Allergy Clin Immunol 2004;114(2):239–47.

16. Simpson A, Tan VYF, Winn J, et al. Beyond atopy: multiple patterns of sensitization in relation to asthma in a birth cohort study. Am J Respir Crit Care Med 2010;181(11):1200–6.

17. Fitzpatrick AM, Teague WG. Severe asthma in children: insights from the National Heart, Lung, and Blood Institute's Severe Asthma Research Program. Pediatr Allergy Immunol Pulmonol 2010;23(2):131–8.

18. Busse WW, Morgan WJ, Gergen PJ, et al. Randomized trial of omalizumab (Anti-IgE) for asthma in inner-city children. N Engl J Med 2011;364(11):1005–15.

19. Yunginger JW, Reed CE, O'Connell EJ, et al. A community-based study of the epidemiology of asthma: incidence rates, 1964–1983. Am Rev Respir Dis 1992;146(4):888–94.

20. Lim RH, Kobzik L, Dahl M. Risk for asthma in offspring of asthmatic mothers versus fathers: a meta-analysis. PLoS One 2010;5(4):e10134. Stanojevic S, ed.

21. Jaakkola J, Ahmed P, Ieromnimon A, et al. Preterm delivery and asthma: a systematic review and meta-analysis. J Allergy Clin Immunol 2006;118(4):823–30.

22. Egan KB, Ettinger AS, Bracken MB. Childhood body mass index and subsequent physician-diagnosed asthma: a systematic review and meta-analysis of prospective cohort studies. BMC Pediatr 2013;13(1):121.

23. Forno E, Celedon JC. Asthma and ethnic minorities: socioeconomic status and beyond. Curr Opin Allergy Clin Immunol 2009;9(2):154–60. Available at: http://www.ncbi.nlm.nih.gov/pubmed/19326508. Accessed May 29, 2018.

24. Gupta RS, Zhang X, Sharp LK, et al. Geographic variability in childhood asthma prevalence in Chicago. J Allergy Clin Immunol 2008;121(3):639–45.e1.

25. Wright RJ, Subramanian SV. Advancing a multilevel framework for epidemiologic research on asthma disparities. Chest 2007;132(5 Suppl):757S–69S.

26. Fitzpatrick AM, Teague WG, Meyers DA, et al. Heterogeneity of severe asthma in childhood: confirmation by cluster analysis of children in the National Institutes of Health/National Heart, Lung, and Blood Institute Severe Asthma Research Program. J Allergy Clin Immunol 2011;127(2):382–9.e1-13.

27. Williams DR, Sternthal M, Wright RJ. Social determinants: taking the social context of asthma seriously. Pediatrics 2009;123(Supplement 3):S174–84.

28. Gold DR, Wright R. Population disparities in asthma. Annu Rev Public Health 2005;26(1):89–113.

29. Federico MJ, Liu AH. Overcoming childhood asthma disparities of the inner-city poor. Pediatr Clin North Am 2003;50(3):655–75, vii. http://www.ncbi.nlm.nih.gov/pubmed/12877240. Accessed May 29, 2018.

30. Leong AB, Ramsey CD, Celedón JC. The challenge of asthma in minority populations. Clin Rev Allergy Immunol 2012;43(1–2):156–83.

31. Busse WW, Mitchell H. Addressing issues of asthma in inner-city children. J Allergy Clin Immunol 2007;119(1):43–9.

32. Wright RJ. Perinatal stress and early life programming of lung structure and function. Biol Psychol 2010;84(1):46–56.

33. van de Loo KFE, van Gelder MMHJ, Roukema J, et al. Prenatal maternal psychological stress and childhood asthma and wheezing: a meta-analysis. Eur Respir J 2016;47(1):133–46.

34. Hartwig IRV, Sly PD, Schmidt LA, et al. Prenatal adverse life events increase the risk for atopic diseases in children, which is enhanced in the absence of a maternal atopic predisposition. J Allergy Clin Immunol 2014;134(1):160–9.

35. Thorburn AN, McKenzie CI, Shen S, et al. Evidence that asthma is a developmental origin disease influenced by maternal diet and bacterial metabolites. Nat Commun 2015;6(1):7320.

36. Moore WC, Meyers DA, Wenzel SE, et al. Identification of asthma phenotypes using cluster analysis in the severe asthma research program. Am J Respir Crit Care Med 2010;181(4):315–23.

37. O'Toole J, Mikulic L, Kaminsky DA. Epidemiology and pulmonary physiology of severe asthma. Immunol Allergy Clin North Am 2016;36(3):425–38.

38. Mauad T, Silva LFF, Santos MA, et al. Abnormal alveolar attachments with decreased elastic fiber content in distal lung in fatal asthma. Am J Respir Crit Care Med 2004;170(8):857–62.

39. Payne DNR, Rogers AV, Adelroth E, et al. Early thickening of the reticular basement membrane in children with difficult asthma. Am J Respir Crit Care Med 2003;167(1):78–82.

40. Tillie-Leblond I, de Blic J, Jaubert F, et al. Airway remodeling is correlated with obstruction in children with severe asthma. Allergy 2008;63(5):533–41.

41. Dolhnikoff M, da Silva LFF, de Araujo BB, et al. The outer wall of small airways is a major site of remodeling in fatal asthma. J Allergy Clin Immunol 2009;123(5): 1090–7, 1097.e1.

42. Gibson PG, Norzila MZ, Fakes K, et al. Pattern of airway inflammation and its determinants in children with acute severe asthma. Pediatr Pulmonol 1999;28(4): 261–70. Available at: http://www.ncbi.nlm.nih.gov/pubmed/10497375. Accessed May 4, 2018.

43. Andersson CK, Adams A, Nagakumar P, et al. Intraepithelial neutrophils in pediatric severe asthma are associated with better lung function. J Allergy Clin Immunol 2017;139(6):1819–29.e11.

44. Jackson DJ, Gangnon RE, Evans MD, et al. Wheezing rhinovirus illnesses in early life predict asthma development in high-risk children. Am J Respir Crit Care Med 2008;178(7):667–72.

45. Wenzel SE, Schwartz LB, Langmack EL, et al. Evidence that severe asthma can be divided pathologically into two inflammatory subtypes with distinct physiologic and clinical characteristics. Am J Respir Crit Care Med 1999;160(3):1001–8.

46. Brown SD, Brown LA, Stephenson S, et al. Characterization of a high TNF-α phenotype in children with moderate-to-severe asthma. J Allergy Clin Immunol 2015;135(6):1651–4.

47. O'Brien CE, Tsirilakis K, Santiago MT, et al. Heterogeneity of lower airway inflammation in children with severe-persistent asthma. Pediatr Pulmonol 2015;50(12): 1200–4.

48. Bossley CJ, Fleming L, Gupta A, et al. Pediatric severe asthma is characterized by eosinophilia and remodeling without T(H)2 cytokines. J Allergy Clin Immunol 2012;129(4):974–82.e13.

49. Hansbro PM, Starkey MR, Mattes J, et al. Pulmonary immunity during respiratory infections in early life and the development of severe asthma. Ann Am Thorac Soc 2014;11(Supplement 5):S297–302.

50. Hilty M, Burke C, Pedro H, et al. Disordered microbial communities in asthmatic airways. PLoS One 2010;5(1):e8578. Neyrolles O, ed.

51. Jartti T, Gern JE. Role of viral infections in the development and exacerbation of asthma in children. J Allergy Clin Immunol 2017;140(4):895–906.

52. Bacharier LB, Strunk RC, Mauger D, et al. Classifying asthma severity in children: mismatch between symptoms, medication use, and lung function. Am J Respir Crit Care Med 2004;170(4):426–32.

53. Normansell R, Walker S, Milan SJ, et al. Omalizumab for asthma in adults and children. Cochrane Database Syst Rev 2014;(1):CD003559.

54. (* NEW) 2018 GINA Report: global strategy for asthma management and prevention | Global Initiative for Asthma – GINA. Available at: http://ginasthma. org/2018-gina-report-global-strategy-for-asthma-management-and-prevention/. Accessed May 1, 2018.

55. Chang TS, Lemanske RF, Mauger DT, et al. Childhood asthma clusters and response to therapy in clinical trials. J Allergy Clin Immunol 2014;133(2):363–9.

56. Wenzel SE. Asthma phenotypes: the evolution from clinical to molecular approaches. Nat Med 2012;18(5):716–25.

57. Reddel H. Emerging concepts in evidence-based asthma management. Semin Respir Crit Care Med 2018;39(01):82–90.

58. Robinson DS, Campbell DA, Durham SR, et al. Systematic assessment of difficult-to-treat asthma. Eur Respir J 2003;22(3):478–83.

59. Barsky EE, Giancola LM, Baxi SN, et al. A practical approach to severe asthma in children. Ann Am Thorac Soc 2018;15(4):399–408.

60. Tantisira KG, Fuhlbrigge AL, Tonascia J, et al. Bronchodilation and bronchoconstriction: predictors of future lung function in childhood asthma. J Allergy Clin Immunol 2006;117(6):1264–71.

61. Beydon N, Davis SD, Lombardi E, et al. An official American Thoracic Society/ European Respiratory Society Statement: pulmonary function testing in preschool children. Am J Respir Crit Care Med 2007;175(12):1304–45.

62. Busse WW, Camargo CA, Boushey HA, et al. Expert Panel Report 3: Guidelines for the diagnosis and management of asthma - Summary Report 2007. Washington, DC: US Department of Health and Human Services, National Institutes of Health, National Heart, Lung, and Blood Institute; 2007.

63. Bateman ED, Hurd SS, Barnes PJ, et al. Global strategy for asthma management and prevention: GINA executive summary. Eur Respir J 2008;31(1):143–78.

64. Chung KF. Diagnosis and management of severe asthma. Semin Respir Crit Care Med 2018;39(01):091–9.

65. Guidelines for the diagnosis and management of asthma (EPR-3) | National Heart, Lung, and Blood Institute (NHLBI). Available at: https://www.nhlbi.nih. gov/health-topics/guidelines-for-diagnosis-management-of-asthma. Accessed May 20, 2018.

66. Bossley CJ, Fleming L, Ullmann N, et al. Assessment of corticosteroid response in pediatric patients with severe asthma by using a multidomain approach. J Allergy Clin Immunol 2016;138(2):413–20.e6.

67. Rodrigo GJ, Neffen H. Efficacy and safety of tiotropium in school-age children with moderate-to-severe symptomatic asthma: a systematic review. Pediatr Allergy Immunol 2017;28(6):573–8.

68. Corren J, Kavati A, Ortiz B, et al. Efficacy and safety of omalizumab in children and adolescents with moderate-to-severe asthma: a systematic literature review. Allergy Asthma Proc 2017;38(4):250–63.

69. Esquivel A, Busse WW, Calatroni A, et al. Effects of omalizumab on rhinovirus infections, illnesses, and exacerbations of asthma. Am J Respir Crit Care Med 2017;196(8):985–92.

70. Teach SJ, Gill MA, Togias A, et al. Preseasonal treatment with either omalizumab or an inhaled corticosteroid boost to prevent fall asthma exacerbations. J Allergy Clin Immunol 2015;136(6):1476–85.

71. Pavord ID, Korn S, Howarth P, et al. Mepolizumab for severe eosinophilic asthma (DREAM): a multicentre, double-blind, placebo-controlled trial. Lancet 2012;380(9842):651–9.

72. Bel EH, Wenzel SE, Thompson PJ, et al. Oral glucocorticoid-sparing effect of mepolizumab in eosinophilic asthma. N Engl J Med 2014;371(13):1189–97.

73. Ortega HG, Liu MC, Pavord ID, et al. Mepolizumab treatment in patients with severe eosinophilic asthma. N Engl J Med 2014;371(13):1198–207.

74. FitzGerald JM, Bleecker ER, Nair P, et al. Benralizumab, an anti-interleukin-5 receptor α monoclonal antibody, as add-on treatment for patients with severe, uncontrolled, eosinophilic asthma (CALIMA): a randomised, double-blind, placebo-controlled phase 3 trial. Lancet 2016;388(10056):2128–41.

75. Bleecker ER, FitzGerald JM, Chanez P, et al. Efficacy and safety of benralizumab for patients with severe asthma uncontrolled with high-dosage inhaled corticosteroids and long-acting β2-agonists (SIROCCO): a randomised, multicentre, placebo-controlled phase 3 trial. Lancet 2016;388(10056):2115–27.

76. Rabe KF, Nair P, Brusselle G, et al. Efficacy and safety of dupilumab in glucocorticoid-dependent severe asthma. N Engl J Med 2018. https://doi.org/10.1056/NEJMoa1804093.

77. Castro M, Corren J, Pavord ID, et al. Dupilumab efficacy and safety in moderate-to-severe uncontrolled asthma. N Engl J Med 2018. https://doi.org/10.1056/NEJMoa1804092.

78. Centers for Disease Control and Prevention. National Center for Environmental Health, Division of Environmental Hazards and Health Effects, Centers for Disease Control and Prevention, Asthma Surveillance Data. Available at: https://www.cdc.gov/asthma/asthmadata.htm. Accessed 2016.

79. Zein JG, Udeh BL, Teague WG, et al. Impact of age and sex on outcomes and hospital cost of acute asthma in the United States, 2011-2012. PLoS One 2016; 11(6). https://doi.org/10.1371/journal.pone.0157301.

80. Gupta R, Margevicius S, DeBoer M, et al. Children with severe asthma are likely to become less severe during adolescence: preliminary results of the SARP III pediatric longitudinal study. Am Thorac Soc Int Meet 2018;A7806. Available at: https://www.atsjournals.org/doi/abs/10.1164/ajrccmconference.2018.197.1_MeetingAbstracts.A7806.

81. McGeachie MJ, Yates KP, Zhou X, et al. Patterns of growth and decline in lung function in persistent childhood asthma. N Engl J Med 2016;374(19):1842–52.

82. Vonk JM, Jongepier H, Panhuysen CIM, et al. Risk factors associated with the presence of irreversible airflow limitation and reduced transfer coefficient in patients with asthma after 26 years of follow up. Thorax 2003;58(4):322–7. Available at: http://www.ncbi.nlm.nih.gov/pubmed/12668795. Accessed May 5, 2018.

83. Tai A, Tran H, Roberts M, et al. Outcomes of childhood asthma to the age of 50 years. J Allergy Clin Immunol 2014;133(6):1572–8.e3.

84. Tai A, Tran H, Roberts M, et al. The association between childhood asthma and adult chronic obstructive pulmonary disease. Thorax 2014;69(9):805–10.

85. Phipatanakul W, Mauger DT, Sorkness RL, et al. Effects of age and disease severity on systemic corticosteroid responses in asthma. Am J Respir Crit Care Med 2017;195(11):1439–48.

86. Bui DS, Lodge CJ, Burgess JA, et al. Childhood predictors of lung function trajectories and future COPD risk: a prospective cohort study from the first to the sixth decade of life. Lancet Respir Med 2018. https://doi.org/10.1016/S2213-2600(18)30100-0.

87. Akinbami LJ, Moorman JE, Garbe PL, et al. Status of childhood asthma in the United States, 1980–2007. Pediatrics 2009;123(Supplement 3):S131–45.

88. Akinbami LJ, Schoendorf KC. Trends in childhood asthma: prevalence, health care utilization, and mortality. Pediatrics 2002;110(2 Pt 1):315–22.
89. Gruchalla RS, Sampson HA, Matsui E, et al. Asthma morbidity among inner-city adolescents receiving guidelines-based therapy: role of predictors in the setting of high adherence. J Allergy Clin Immunol 2009;124(2):213–21.e1.
90. Pongracic JA, Krouse RZ, Babineau DC, et al. Distinguishing characteristics of difficult-to-control asthma in inner-city children and adolescents. J Allergy Clin Immunol 2016;138(4):1030–41.
91. Liu AH, Babineau DC, Krouse RZ, et al. Pathways through which asthma risk factors contribute to asthma severity in inner-city children. J Allergy Clin Immunol 2016;138(4):1042–50.
92. Beck AF, Simmons JM, Huang B, et al. Geomedicine: area-based socioeconomic measures for assessing risk of hospital reutilization among children admitted for asthma. Am J Public Health 2012;102(12):2308–14.
93. Price JH, Khubchandani J, McKinney M, et al. Racial/ethnic disparities in chronic diseases of youths and access to health care in the United States. Biomed Res Int 2013;2013:1–12.
94. Kattan M, Mitchell H, Eggleston P, et al. Characteristics of inner-city children with asthma: the National Cooperative Inner-City Asthma Study. Pediatr Pulmonol 1997;24(4):253–62.
95. Rosa MJ, Lee AG, Wright RJ. Evidence establishing a link between prenatal and early-life stress and asthma development. Curr Opin Allergy Clin Immunol 2018; 18(2):1.
96. Beck AF, Huang B, Simmons JM, et al. Role of financial and social hardships in asthma racial disparities. Pediatrics 2014;133(3):431–9.
97. Morgan WJ, Crain EF, Gruchalla RS, et al. Results of a home-based environmental intervention among urban children with asthma. N Engl J Med 2004; 351(11):1068–80.
98. Leas BF, D'Anci KE, Apter AJ, et al. Effectiveness of indoor allergen reduction in asthma management: A systematic review. J Allergy Clin Immunol 2018;141(5): 1854–69.
99. Permaul P, Phipatanakul W. School environmental intervention programs. J Allergy Clin Immunol Pract 2018;6(1):22–9.
100. Al Aloola NA, Naik-Panvelkar P, Nissen L, et al. Asthma interventions in primary schools–a review. J Asthma 2014;51(8):779–98.
101. Carpenter LM, Lachance L, Wilkin M, et al. Sustaining school-based asthma interventions through policy and practice change. J Sch Health 2013;83(12): 859–66.
102. Beck AF, Klein MD, Schaffzin JK, et al. Identifying and treating a substandard housing cluster using a medical-legal partnership. Pediatrics 2012;130(5): 831–8.
103. Klein MD, Beck AF, Henize AW, et al. Doctors and lawyers collaborating to HeLP Children—: outcomes from a successful partnership between professions. J Health Care Poor Underserved 2013;24(3):1063–73.
104. Raphael JL, Colvin JD. More than wheezing: incorporating social determinants into public policy to improve asthma outcomes in children. Pediatr Res 2017; 81(1):2–3.

Inner-City Asthma in Childhood

Amaziah T. Coleman, MD[a,b,*], Stephen J. Teach, MD, MPH[b,c],
William J. Sheehan, MD[a,b]

KEYWORDS

- Inner-city • Asthma • Disparities • Children

KEY POINTS

- Inner cities include high-risk vulnerable populations of children with asthma.
- Multiple risk factors contribute to morbidity and mortality in inner-city pediatric asthma.
- Environmental and medical interventions that target risk factors have been successful in improving outcomes.

INTRODUCTION

Merriam-Webster defines an inner city as "the usually older, poorer, and more densely populated central section of a city."[1] Historically, the inner cities of major metropolitan areas within the United States have been populated by minority residents,[2] many of whom live in poverty. Asthma is the most common chronic disease of childhood in general; however, asthma also exerts a particularly heavy burden on children living in inner cities.[3,4] In this review, we discuss the epidemiology of asthma in the inner city. We examine both intrinsic and extrinsic contributing factors, including race and ethnicity, prematurity, obesity, specific aeroallergens, pollutants, socioeconomic status, poverty, and psychosocial factors. Finally, we review environmental and medical interventions specific to the management of asthma in the inner city.

EPIDEMIOLOGY

The prevalence of asthma in inner-city populations remains disproportionately high compared with non-urban areas. Typical rates of asthma prevalence among US

Disclosure Statement: The authors have no commercial or financial conflicts of interest.
[a] Division of Allergy and Immunology, Department of Pediatrics, Children's National Health System, 111 Michigan Avenue Northwest, Washington, DC 20010, USA; [b] George Washington University School of Medicine and Health Sciences, Washington, DC, USA; [c] Division of Emergency Medicine, Department of Pediatrics, Children's National Health System, 111 Michigan Avenue Northwest, Washington, DC 20010, USA
* Corresponding author. Children's National Health System, 111 Michigan Avenue Northwest, Washington, DC 20010.
E-mail address: acoleman2@childrensnational.org

children are estimated to be approximately 8% with rates in the inner city up to 28%.[5,6] Overall childhood asthma prevalence seems to have plateaued this decade; however, there remains an increasing prevalence among poor children.[5] Keet and colleagues[7] demonstrated that the high prevalence of asthma in inner cities is not necessarily due to specifically living in an urban neighborhood, but instead may be related to demographic factors such as race, ethnicity, and lower household income. Likewise, a more recent study showed that after controlling for demographic factors, inner-city residence was not associated with an increased asthma prevalence. It was associated with significantly more asthma morbidity, including increased asthma-related emergency department visits and hospitalizations.[8] Multiple studies have similarly shown increased asthma morbidity among inner-city children.[8,9]

INTRINSIC RISK FACTORS
Race and Ethnicity

Evidence has shown that race and ethnicity are contributing factors to asthma disparities. A nationwide health survey linked to census information identified black children and Puerto Ricans of Hispanic ethnicity as independently at higher risk for current asthma among children.[7] In the recent literature, the prevalence of current asthma in black children is twice the prevalence in white children.[10] It is often hypothesized that asthma may be underdiagnosed in certain inner-city minority populations owing to a variety of factors, including concerns of access to care; however, there is evidence to the contrary. Akinbami and colleagues[11] demonstrated that, among symptomatic children, minority children were as or more likely to be diagnosed with asthma than non-Hispanic white children, even after adjusting for the increased severity of wheezing in the minority children. Among Hispanic children, there are varying rates of asthma prevalence with children of Puerto Rican ethnicity having the highest rates that are 2.4 times increased compared with matched white children.[12,13] Interestingly, disparities in asthma morbidity are even seen within children of a similar heritage. One study in children of Caribbean descent living in the inner city found that Puerto Rican children had significantly greater asthma morbidity in the previous year when compared with Afro-Caribbean children; however, there were no differences in spirometry between the 2 groups.[14] In general, emergency department use in Hispanic children with asthma is twice as frequent as in white children with asthma.[10] Additional trends in asthma morbidity are also associated with race. Akinbami and colleagues[15] found that race was an inherent risk factor for worse pediatric asthma outcomes with black children being 7 times more likely to die from asthma, 3 times more likely to be hospitalized for asthma, and more than 2 times more likely to require a visit to the emergency department for asthma when compared with white children.

Prematurity

Premature birth is a recognized risk factor for asthma development in young children and rates of prematurity are increased among inner-city, low-income, and minority neighborhoods.[16] Extreme preterm birth at 23 to 27 weeks of gestation is associated with an even greater increased risk for developing asthma.[17] Non-Hispanic black mothers have disproportionately higher rates of premature deliveries and low birthweight infants.[18,19] Martin and Osterman[20] reported a 60% higher rate of premature birth in black infants compared with children of white or Asian/Pacific Islander descent. Additional studies in low-income populations support prematurity as a risk factor for the development of asthma later in childhood and also identify low birth weight as an associated risk factor for asthma in this population.[21]

Obesity

Childhood obesity is more common in inner-city populations. Previous studies have shown 24% to 29% childhood obesity prevalence in inner-city children compared with 17% nationally.[22,23] This may be related to obesity being more prevalent in certain races and ethnicities. A study by Vo and colleagues[24] examined the relationship among weight, ethnicity, and spirometric values in children with asthma living in the inner-city Bronx, New York. Investigators found that black and Hispanic children were more likely to be overweight or obese than white children. The forced expiratory volume in 1 second (FEV_1)/forced vital capacity ratio was lower in overweight and obese black and Hispanic children. A lower FEV_1/forced vital capacity ratio was associated only with obesity, not being overweight, in white children with asthma. Jensen and colleagues[25] reported that diet-induced weight loss in obese children with asthma resulted in improved lung function and asthma control.

EXTRINSIC RISK FACTORS
Aeroallergens

Pests (cockroaches and mice)
For decades, cockroach and mouse allergens have been well-documented to be implicated in the inner-city asthma problem. Older homes in multiunit buildings with poor upkeep provide the ideal breeding ground for cockroaches and mice. Cockroach allergen is commonly found in inner-city homes and up to 80% of inner-city children have cockroach sensitization.[26] The combination of sensitization and exposure to cockroach has been associated with an increased asthma morbidity in these children.[27] Similarly, mouse allergen exposure is a frequent problem in the inner city and up to one-half of children living in urban neighborhoods are sensitized to mouse allergen.[28–32] Exposure to mouse allergen is a significant source of higher risk of asthma morbidity in children known to have sensitization.[29,30] In fact, Ahluwalia and colleagues[29] have demonstrated that, in urban areas with high levels of both mouse and cockroach allergens, mouse allergen was more strongly and consistently associated with asthma morbidity when compared with cockroach allergen. Outside of the home, cockroach and mouse allergens have also been problematic in urban school settings with classroom-specific mouse allergen exposure in inner-city schools associated with increased asthma symptoms and decreased spirometry in asthmatic students.[33,34]

Molds
Poor conditions in urban homes can lead to a wall cracks, water leaks, indoor dampness, and fungal spores. O'Connor and colleagues[35] discovered that mold-sensitized children with asthma living in inner-city environments were exposed to airborne fungi in both indoor and outdoor air. It was then demonstrated that urban children with asthma exposed to higher levels of indoor fungi had significant increases in unscheduled visits for asthma, even after controlling for outdoor fungal levels.[36]

Pollens
Factors in urban areas may facilitate susceptibility to increased pollen production. For example, Ziska and colleagues[37] noted that, when compared with rural environments, urban environments in the United States had higher temperatures and carbon dioxide production that was associated with ragweed plants growing faster, flowering earlier, and producing more pollen. This is supported by European data demonstrating an increasing trend in yearly amount of airborne pollen that was more pronounced in urban areas.[38]

Pollutants

Indoor pollutants

Two of the most significant indoor pollutants include environmental tobacco smoke and indoor nitrogen dioxide. Indoor nitrogen dioxide is most commonly emitted from gas stoves. In a multicenter inner-city asthma study, investigators found that almost 90% of urban homes had gas stoves and those homes had high levels of nitrogen dioxide with a median nitrogen dioxide level of 29.8 ppb and 24% of homes with extremely high exposures (>40 ppb).[39] Increased nitrogen dioxide exposure in these inner-city homes was associated with an increased risk for asthma symptoms in non-atopic children.[39] Similarly, Hansel and colleagues[40] evaluated the home environments of preschool children with asthma living in inner-city Baltimore and found a mean concentration of nitrogen dioxide in this population to be 30 ppb with increased indoor nitrogen dioxide levels associated with increased asthma symptoms.

Environmental tobacco exposure

Environmental tobacco exposure is a well-known risk factor for increased asthma that has been well-studied in inner-city children. A recent publication from the Urban Environment and Childhood Asthma (URECA) cohort demonstrated that prenatal exposure to tobacco smoke is associated with increased risk for asthma development.[41] Investigators in the Inner-City Asthma Consortium (ICAC) study developed a conceptual model to explain how 8 risk-factor domains are linked to asthma severity. Results of the study revealed that the environmental tobacco smoke exposure pathway, which linked environmental tobacco smoke exposure and pulmonary physiology with asthma severity, resulted in significant effects on asthma severity.[42]

Outdoor pollutants

Outdoor air pollutants such as outdoor traffic-related emissions like carbon monoxide, nitrogen dioxide, ozone, and particulate matter are associated with increased asthma risk in children.[43–45] Children living in inner city environments have more exposure to outdoor air pollutants owing to living closer to major highways and bus routes.[19,46,47] Investigators in the Childhood Asthma Management Program (CAMP) found that short and long-term exposures to outdoor air pollutants such as carbon monoxide, ozone, nitrogen dioxide, and sulfur dioxide were associated with impaired lung function in children with asthma.[48]

Socioeconomic Status and Poverty

Poverty is both common in inner cities and a known risk factor for increased asthma prevalence. A 2012 National Health Interview Survey reported a 13% asthma prevalence rate in children living below the federal poverty level compared with an 8% asthma prevalence rate in children living above the federal poverty level.[43,49] This finding may be related to race and ethnicity also being a risk factor as described elsewhere in this article. For example, in 2013, it was noted that 36.9% of African American children and 30.4% of Hispanic children were living in poverty, compared with only 10.7% of non-Hispanic White children.[50] Investigators in the inner-city URECA birth cohort identified poverty as a risk factor for recurrent wheeze.[43,51] In a national epidemiologic study of more than 23,000 children, Keet and colleagues[7] reported that poverty was an independent risk factor when controlling for asthma, race, ethnicity, and urban residence.

Psychosocial Factors

Psychosocial factors and social determinants of health have been shown to influence asthma morbidity in inner-city children. A study of caregiver's perception of neighborhood safety found that children living in the inner city had increased asthma morbidity when their caregivers felt that the neighborhood was unsafe.[52] Shams and colleagues[53] demonstrated that in inner-city black adolescents with persistent asthma, anxiety was associated with poor asthma control, impaired quality of life, insomnia, and increased emergency department visits for asthma. Even maternal stress and depression have been associated with recurrent wheezing at 3 years of age in inner-city populations.[54] Additionally, higher daily stress is associated with increased childhood asthma-related emergency service use.[55]

INTERVENTIONS AND MANAGEMENT

In 2012, the President's Task Force on Environmental Health Risks and Safety Risks to Children published the Coordinated Federal Action Plan to Reduce Racial and Ethnic Asthma Disparities.[56] This action plan combines the collaboration of a broad spectrum of federal agencies that constitute the Asthma Disparities Working Group. The action plan has identified 4 strategies to address the preventable factors leading to asthma disparities. These 4 strategies include:

1. Reducing barriers to the implementation of guidelines-based asthma management;
2. Enhancing the capacity to deliver integrated, comprehensive asthma care to children in communities with racial and ethnic asthma disparities;
3. Improving the capacity to identify the children most impacted by asthma disparities; and
4. Accelerating efforts to identify and test interventions that may prevent the onset of asthma among ethnic and racial minority children.

The report identifies the need for integrated, multimodal approaches to addressing racial and ethnic disparities in asthma and provides a framework for intervention strategies. Several of the action plan's strategies specifically address priority actions that are risk factors for inner-city asthma, including reducing environmental exposures in homes and schools, protecting children from health risks associated with exposure to air pollutants, and decreasing exposure to environmental tobacco smoke.[56]

Additional studies assessing home management of asthma in the inner city from the perspective of minority children have identified education and self-management support, environmental control measures, housing resources, access to smoking cessation interventions, and psychosocial support as a suggested multipronged approach to management.[57]

Environmental Interventions

Several studies have targeted environmental interventions to reduce indoor allergen exposure as a treatment regimen. Depending on the specific population and location, children are more likely to be exposed to particular allergens. Interventions targeting these allergens have been studied with various approaches.[28]

In a seminal study, Morgan and colleagues[58] demonstrated that an individualized, home-based, comprehensive environmental intervention decreased childhood exposures to cockroach and dust mites allergens resulting in reduced asthma morbidity in inner-city children with atopic asthma. In a more recent study, Rabito and colleagues[59] used a simpler approach of targeted cockroach bait insecticides, which resulted in sustained cockroach elimination and was associated with improved asthma outcomes. For areas of high cockroach infestation, this single allergen intervention may be an alternative to multifaceted interventions.

In addition to cockroach elimination strategies, interventions to reduce mouse allergen exposure have been investigated in the inner city. Mouse allergen reduction efforts typically rely on integrated pest management, which consists of a multifaceted approach that includes vigorous cleaning, sealing of holes and cracks, disposal or putting away of food, mouse traps, and application of rodenticide.[60] Integrated pest management is usually done by professional pest control services, but includes education for residents to maintain a beneficial environment long after the intervention. Pongracic and colleagues[61] demonstrated that rodent-specific environmental interventions were able to reduce home mouse allergen levels and improve clinical outcomes in inner-city children with asthma.[62] Alternatively, DiMango and colleagues[63] implemented an individualized allergen intervention that was able to decrease allergen levels, but did not result in a decrease in asthma medication use between intervention and control groups. More recently, the Mouse Allergen and Asthma Intervention Trial (MAAIT) compared professional integrated pest management with education to education alone in inner-city children with documented mouse exposure and mouse sensitization.[62] The MAAIT trial did not find a significant difference in asthma symptoms days between the 2 treatment groups because many participants in both arms experienced a significant reduction in mouse allergen exposure and symptomatology.[62] This finding indicates the success of education alone in this particular trial. However, across both groups, there was a dose–response relationship between mouse allergen reduction and improvements in asthma.[62] These studies indicate that successful allergen reductions in the inner city can lead to improved asthma outcomes. Future studies may focus on the most efficient and effective ways to achieve these positive outcomes in the inner city.

Medical Management

In 2007, the National Heart, Lung and Blood Institute of the National Institutes of Health published the Expert Panel Report-3, which provides evidence-based guidelines for the diagnosis of and management of asthma. For more than 10 years, the Expert Panel Report-3 has been an effective tool for clinicians treating asthma.[64] The Asthma Control Evaluation (ACE) trial was developed by the ICAC and implemented from 2002 to 2008. This study showed that guidelines-based management for asthma in an inner-city population of adolescents and young adults was adequate for asthma control. Investigators also discovered that the addition of measuring fraction of exhaled nitric oxide to modify treatment did not result in better clinical control of asthma.[65] During the ACE trial, 71% to 78% of both control and intervention group participants maintained asthma control. This level of adherence to guidelines-based care can be more challenging to achieve outside the clinical trial setting.[65]

Additional approaches, such as immunomodulatory therapies, have become an important tool for asthma management in recent years. Within ICAC, Busse and colleagues[66] showed that adding omalizumab (anti-IgE) to guidelines-based therapy in inner-city children resulted in a decrease in asthma symptom days, a decrease in seasonal peaks in exacerbations, and a decreased need for other controller medications. Based on these results, a second study by the same ICAC group evaluated targeted short-term omalizumab therapy beginning just before the start of the school year and continuing for only 4 months. The researchers found this temporary omalizumab treatment approach for inner-city children was able to significantly decrease autumnal exacerbation rates, particularly among those children with a recent exacerbation.[67]

More recent studies of another immunomodulatory agent, dupilumab (anti-IL4 receptor alpha), has shown its effectiveness in decreasing oral steroid use, the frequency of severe exacerbations, and increasing FEV_1 in steroid-dependent severe asthma.[68] Dupilumab has also been shown to significantly lower the frequency of asthma exacerbations and improve lung function and asthma control in individuals with uncontrolled moderate to severe asthma.[69] Additional studies of dupilumab in the inner-city pediatric population are warranted. Although immunomodulatory therapies such as omalizumab and dupilumab have proven to be effective interventions in asthma management, it is important to remain aware of barriers such as access to care, ability to obtain medications, and adherence to treatment regimens that may make achieving asthma control more difficult in this population.

In the Asthma Phenotypes in Inner-City (APIC) study, researchers uncovered certain factors associated with difficult-to-control pediatric asthma including elevations of circulating blood eosinophils, neutrophils, and certain cytokines (CXCL-1, IL-5, IL-8, IL-17A).[70] Investigators from the study initially showed that FEV_1 bronchodilator responsiveness was the most important distinguishing characteristic between difficult-to-control and easy-to-control asthma in children living in the inner city. Rhinitis severity and atopy were other distinguishing characteristics. Over time, difficult-to-control asthma in this population was associated with increased morbidity.[71] Knowledge of these factors contributing to increased disease severity in inner city children with asthma may guide management and future research directions.

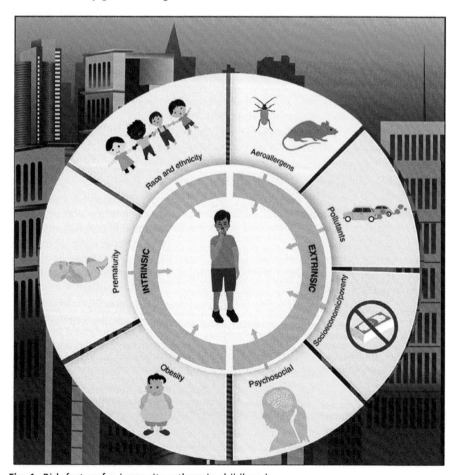

Fig. 1. Risk factors for inner-city asthma in childhood.

SUMMARY

Residing in the inner city is an established and important risk factor for asthma. The prevalence of asthma remains high in the inner city compared with nonurban areas. This prevalence has been shown to be related not only to the inner-city locale, but also to both extrinsic and intrinsic factors, such as race, ethnicity, and a lower household income. Prematurity and obesity are additional intrinsic risk factors that are common in the inner city. Regarding extrinsic inner-city risk factors for childhood asthma, cockroach, mouse, and mold remain the most relevant aeroallergens contributing to disease burden. Indoor pollutants such as nitrogen dioxide and environmental tobacco smoke are common in the inner city and significant risk factors for increased asthma severity. Living in the inner city also exposes children with asthma to more outdoor pollutants such as carbon monoxide, nitrogen dioxide, ozone, and particulate matter. Poverty, stress, and psychosocial factors also contribute to increased morbidity in the inner-city population (**Fig. 1**). With increasing knowledge of risk factors associated with inner-city childhood asthma, investigators and clinicians have been able to implement interventions, including indoor environmental control measures, smoking cessation, and educational and psychological support. Medical interventions based on asthma phenotype have also shown to be beneficial in inner-city childhood asthma. More studies aimed at identifying and targeting risk factors and implementing interventions and therapies will be pertinent for decreasing disparities in this high-risk vulnerable population of children with asthma.

REFERENCES

1. Merriam-Webster. Inner-city. Available at: https://www.merriam-webster.com/dictionary/inner city. Accessed February 2, 2018.
2. Urban settlement. Encyclopedia britannica. Available at: https://www.britannica.com/place/United-States/Impact-of-the-motor-vehicle - ref77981. Accessed February 2, 2018.
3. Weiss KB, Gergen PJ, Crain EF. Inner-city asthma. The epidemiology of an emerging US public health concern. Chest 1992;101(6 Suppl):362S–7S.
4. Togias A, Fenton MJ, Gergen PJ, et al. Asthma in the inner city: the perspective of the National Institute of Allergy and Infectious Diseases. J Allergy Clin Immunol 2010;125(3):540–4.
5. Akinbami LJ, Simon AE, Schoendorf KC. Trends in allergy prevalence among children aged 0-17 years by asthma status, United States, 2001-2013. J Asthma 2016;53(4):356–62.
6. Bryant-Stephens T, West C, Dirl C, et al. Asthma prevalence in Philadelphia: description of two community-based methodologies to assess asthma prevalence in an inner-city population. J Asthma 2012;49(6):581–5.
7. Keet CA, McCormack MC, Pollack CE, et al. Neighborhood poverty, urban residence, race/ethnicity, and asthma: rethinking the inner-city asthma epidemic. J Allergy Clin Immunol 2015;135(3):655–62.
8. Keet CA, Matsui EC, McCormack MC, et al. Urban residence, neighborhood poverty, race/ethnicity, and asthma morbidity among children on Medicaid. J Allergy Clin Immunol 2017;140(3):822–7.
9. Gergen PJ, Teach SJ, Togias A, et al. Reducing exacerbations in the inner city: lessons from the inner-city asthma consortium (ICAC). J Allergy Clin Immunol Pract 2016;4(1):22–6.

10. Akinbami LJ, Moorman JE, Simon AE, et al. Trends in racial disparities for asthma outcomes among children 0 to 17 years, 2001-2010. J Allergy Clin Immunol 2014; 134(3):547–553 e545.

11. Akinbami LJ, Rhodes JC, Lara M. Racial and ethnic differences in asthma diagnosis among children who wheeze. Pediatrics 2005;115(5):1254–60.

12. Carter-Pokras OD, Gergen PJ. Reported asthma among Puerto Rican, Mexican-American, and Cuban children, 1982 through 1984. Am J Public Health 1993; 83(4):580–2.

13. Ledogar RJ, Penchaszadeh A, Garden CC, et al. Asthma and Latino cultures: different prevalence reported among groups sharing the same environment. Am J Public Health 2000;90(6):929–35.

14. Steinberg DM, Serebrisky D, Feldman JM. Asthma in children of Caribbean descent living in the inner-city: comparing Puerto Rican and Afro-Caribbean children. Psychol Health Med 2017;22(6):633–9.

15. Akinbami LJ, Moorman JE, Garbe PL, et al. Status of childhood asthma in the United States, 1980-2007. Pediatrics 2009;123(Suppl 3):S131–45.

16. He H, Butz A, Keet CA, et al. Preterm birth with childhood asthma: the role of degree of prematurity and asthma definitions. Am J Respir Crit Care Med 2015; 192(4):520–3.

17. Crump C, Winkleby MA, Sundquist J, et al. Risk of asthma in young adults who were born preterm: a Swedish national cohort study. Pediatrics 2011;127(4): e913–20.

18. Martin JA, Hamilton BE, Osterman MJ, et al. Births: final data for 2012. Natl Vital Stat Rep 2013;62(9):1–68.

19. Gergen PJ, Togias A. Inner city asthma. Immunol Allergy Clin North Am 2015; 35(1):101–14.

20. Martin JA, Osterman MJ, Centers for Disease Control and Prevention (CDC). Preterm births - United States, 2006 and 2010. MMWR Suppl 2013;62(3):136–8.

21. Dombkowski KJ, Leung SW, Gurney JG. Prematurity as a predictor of childhood asthma among low-income children. Ann Epidemiol 2008;18(4):290–7.

22. Robbins JM, Benson BJ, Esangbedo IC, et al. Childhood obesity in an inner-city primary care population: a longitudinal study. J Natl Med Assoc 2016;108(3): 158–63.

23. Elliott JP, Harrison C, Konopka C, et al. Pharmacist-led screening program for an inner-city pediatric population. J Am Pharm Assoc (2003) 2015;55(4):413–8.

24. Vo P, Makker K, Matta-Arroyo E, et al. The association of overweight and obesity with spirometric values in minority children referred for asthma evaluation. J Asthma 2013;50(1):56–63.

25. Jensen ME, Gibson PG, Collins CE, et al. Diet-induced weight loss in obese children with asthma: a randomized controlled trial. Clin Exp Allergy 2013;43(7): 775–84.

26. Eggleston PA, Rosenstreich D, Lynn H, et al. Relationship of indoor allergen exposure to skin test sensitivity in inner-city children with asthma. J Allergy Clin Immunol 1998;102(4 Pt 1):563–70.

27. Rosenstreich DL, Eggleston P, Kattan M, et al. The role of cockroach allergy and exposure to cockroach allergen in causing morbidity among inner-city children with asthma. N Engl J Med 1997;336(19):1356–63.

28. Ahluwalia SK, Matsui EC. Indoor environmental interventions for furry pet allergens, pest allergens, and mold: looking to the future. J Allergy Clin Immunol Pract 2018;6(1):9–19.

29. Ahluwalia SK, Peng RD, Breysse PN, et al. Mouse allergen is the major allergen of public health relevance in Baltimore City. J Allergy Clin Immunol 2013;132(4): 830–5.e1-2.

30. Torjusen EN, Diette GB, Breysse PN, et al. Dose-response relationships between mouse allergen exposure and asthma morbidity among urban children and adolescents. Indoor Air 2013;23(4):268–74.

31. Matsui EC, Eggleston PA, Buckley TJ, et al. Household mouse allergen exposure and asthma morbidity in inner-city preschool children. Ann Allergy Asthma Immunol 2006;97(4):514–20.

32. Phipatanakul W, Eggleston PA, Wright EC, et al, National Cooperative Inner-City Asthma Study. Mouse allergen. II. The relationship of mouse allergen exposure to mouse sensitization and asthma morbidity in inner-city children with asthma. J Allergy Clin Immunol 2000;106(6):1075–80.

33. Sheehan WJ, Rangsithienchai PA, Muilenberg ML, et al. Mouse allergens in urban elementary schools and homes of children with asthma. Ann Allergy Asthma Immunol 2009;102(2):125–30.

34. Chew GL. Assessment of environmental cockroach allergen exposure. Curr Allergy Asthma Rep 2012;12(5):456–64.

35. O'Connor GT, Walter M, Mitchell H, et al. Airborne fungi in the homes of children with asthma in low-income urban communities: the Inner-City Asthma Study. J Allergy Clin Immunol 2004;114(3):599–606.

36. Pongracic JA, O'Connor GT, Muilenberg ML, et al. Differential effects of outdoor versus indoor fungal spores on asthma morbidity in inner-city children. J Allergy Clin Immunol 2010;125(3):593–9.

37. Ziska LH, Gebhard DE, Frenz DA, et al. Cities as harbingers of climate change: common ragweed, urbanization, and public health. J Allergy Clin Immunol 2003; 111(2):290–5.

38. Ziello C, Sparks TH, Estrella N, et al. Changes to airborne pollen counts across Europe. PLoS One 2012;7(4):e34076.

39. Kattan M, Gergen PJ, Eggleston P, et al. Health effects of indoor nitrogen dioxide and passive smoking on urban asthmatic children. J Allergy Clin Immunol 2007; 120(3):618–24.

40. Hansel NN, Breysse PN, McCormack MC, et al. A longitudinal study of indoor nitrogen dioxide levels and respiratory symptoms in inner-city children with asthma. Environ Health Perspect 2008;116(10):1428–32.

41. O'Connor GT, Lynch SV, Bloomberg GR, et al. Early-life home environment and risk of asthma among inner-city children. J Allergy Clin Immunol 2018;141(4): 1468–75.

42. Liu AH, Babineau DC, Krouse RZ, et al. Pathways through which asthma risk factors contribute to asthma severity in inner-city children. J Allergy Clin Immunol 2016;138(4):1042–50.

43. Milligan KL, Matsui E, Sharma H. Asthma in urban children: epidemiology, environmental risk factors, and the public health domain. Curr Allergy Asthma Rep 2016;16(4):33.

44. Guarnieri M, Balmes JR. Outdoor air pollution and asthma. Lancet 2014; 383(9928):1581–92.

45. Gauderman WJ, Urman R, Avol E, et al. Association of improved air quality with lung development in children. N Engl J Med 2015;372(10):905–13.

46. Ruffin J. A renewed commitment to environmental justice in health disparities research. Am J Public Health 2011;101(Suppl 1):S12–4.

47. Cureton S. Environmental victims: environmental injustice issues that threaten the health of children living in poverty. Rev Environ Health 2011;26(3):141–7.

48. Ierodiakonou D, Zanobetti A, Coull BA, et al. Ambient air pollution, lung function, and airway responsiveness in asthmatic children. J Allergy Clin Immunol 2016; 137(2):390–9.

49. Bloom B, Jones LI, Freeman G. Summary health statistics for U.S. children: National Health Interview Survey, 2012. Vital Health Stat 10 2013;(258):1–81.

50. Department of Health and Human Services, Office of the Assistant Secretary for Planning and Evaluation. Information on poverty and income statistics: a summary of 2014 current population survey data. Washington, DC: ASPE Office of Human Services Policy; 2014. p. 1–9. Available at: https://aspe.hhs.gov/report/information-poverty-and-income-statistics-summary-2014-current-population-survey-data.

51. Lynch SV, Wood RA, Boushey H, et al. Effects of early-life exposure to allergens and bacteria on recurrent wheeze and atopy in urban children. J Allergy Clin Immunol 2014;134(3):593–601.e12.

52. Kopel LS, Gaffin JM, Ozonoff A, et al. Perceived neighborhood safety and asthma morbidity in the school inner-city asthma study. Pediatr Pulmonol 2015;50(1): 17–24.

53. Shams MR, Bruce AC, Fitzpatrick AM. Anxiety contributes to poorer asthma outcomes in inner-city black adolescents. J Allergy Clin Immunol Pract 2018;6(1): 227–35.

54. Ramratnam SK, Visness CM, Jaffee KF, et al. Relationships among maternal stress and depression, type 2 responses, and recurrent wheezing at age 3 years in low-income urban families. Am J Respir Crit Care Med 2017;195(5):674–81.

55. Bellin MH, Collins KS, Osteen P, et al. Characterization of stress in low-income, inner-city mothers of children with poorly controlled asthma. J Urban Health 2017;94(6):814–23.

56. Coordinated federal action plan to reduce racial and ethnic asthma disparities. Available at: http://www.epa.gov/childrenstaskforce/federal_asthma_disparities_action_plan.pdf. Accessed May 1, 2018.

57. Bellin MH, Newsome A, Land C, et al. Asthma home management in the inner-city: what can the children teach us? J Pediatr Health Care 2017;31(3):362–71.

58. Morgan WJ, Crain EF, Gruchalla RS, et al. Results of a home-based environmental intervention among urban children with asthma. N Engl J Med 2004; 351(11):1068–80.

59. Rabito FA, Carlson JC, He H, et al. A single intervention for cockroach control reduces cockroach exposure and asthma morbidity in children. J Allergy Clin Immunol 2017;140(2):565–70.

60. Phipatanakul W, Matsui E, Portnoy J, et al. Environmental assessment and exposure reduction of rodents: a practice parameter. Ann Allergy Asthma Immunol 2012;109(6):375–87.

61. Pongracic JA, Visness CM, Gruchalla RS, et al. Effect of mouse allergen and rodent environmental intervention on asthma in inner-city children. Ann Allergy Asthma Immunol 2008;101(1):35–41.

62. Matsui EC, Perzanowski M, Peng RD, et al. Effect of an integrated pest management intervention on asthma symptoms among mouse-sensitized children and adolescents with asthma: a randomized clinical trial. JAMA 2017;317(10): 1027–36.

63. DiMango E, Serebrisky D, Narula S, et al. Individualized household allergen intervention lowers allergen level but not asthma medication use: a randomized controlled trial. J Allergy Clin Immunol Pract 2016;4(4):671–679 e674.
64. Expert Panel Report 3. Guidelines for the diagnosis and management of asthma 2007. Available at: https://www.nhlbi.nih.gov/sites/default/files/media/docs/asthgdln_1.pdf. Accessed April 5, 2018.
65. Szefler SJ, Mitchell H, Sorkness CA, et al. Management of asthma based on exhaled nitric oxide in addition to guideline-based treatment for inner-city adolescents and young adults: a randomised controlled trial. Lancet 2008;372(9643): 1065–72.
66. Busse WW, Morgan WJ, Gergen PJ, et al. Randomized trial of omalizumab (anti-IgE) for asthma in inner-city children. N Engl J Med 2011;364(11):1005–15.
67. Teach SJ, Gill MA, Togias A, et al. Preseasonal treatment with either omalizumab or an inhaled corticosteroid boost to prevent fall asthma exacerbations. J Allergy Clin Immunol 2015;136(6):1476–85.
68. Rabe KF, Nair P, Brusselle G, et al. Efficacy and safety of dupilumab in glucocorticoid-dependent severe asthma. N Engl J Med 2018;378(26):2475–85.
69. Castro M, Corren J, Pavord ID, et al. Dupilumab efficacy and safety in moderate-to-severe uncontrolled asthma. N Engl J Med 2018;378(26):2486–96.
70. Brown KR, Krouse RZ, Calatroni A, et al. Endotypes of difficult-to-control asthma in inner-city African American children. PLoS One 2017;12(7):e0180778.
71. Pongracic JA, Krouse RZ, Babineau DC, et al. Distinguishing characteristics of difficult-to-control asthma in inner-city children and adolescents. J Allergy Clin Immunol 2016;138(4):1030–41.

Asthma in Schools
How School-Based Partnerships Improve Pediatric Asthma Care

Sujani Kakumanu, MD[a],*, Robert F. Lemanske Jr, MD[b,c]

KEYWORDS

• Asthma • Schools • Asthma action plans • Circle of support • Asthma education

KEY POINTS

• Partnerships among families, clinicians, and school nurses, centered on the child, establish a circle of support to facilitate asthma care.
• Asthma management plans, including individualized asthma action plans, are fundamental tools in coordinating asthma care with schools.
• Comprehensive asthma education and programs that remediate environmental asthma triggers empower schools to provide safe school environments for children with asthma.

BACKGROUND

In the United States, asthma is a leading chronic health condition in children, affecting 1 in 12 children nationwide.[1] Childhood asthma continues to be associated with significant morbidity and high rates of school absenteeism, particularly in children of low socioeconomic status. Reducing the disparity between children with asthma and healthy children will require extending pediatric asthma care beyond the traditional clinic and hospital settings and building effective health partnerships with the community and schools.

Recent data have shown that asthma continues to affect 6 million school-aged children with approximately half of these children experiencing asthma attacks each year.[1] Encouraging data from the Centers for Disease Control and Prevention (CDC)

The authors have no pertinent commercial or financial disclosures to report.
[a] Department of Medicine, University of Wisconsin School of Medicine and Public Health, William S. Middleton Veterans Memorial Hospital, 600 Highland Avenue CSC 9988, Madison, WI 53792, USA; [b] Department of Pediatrics, Institute for Clinical and Translational Research, University of Wisconsin School of Medicine and Public Health, 4235 HSLC, 750 Highland Avenue, Madison, WI 53705, USA; [c] Department of Medicine, Institute for Clinical and Translational Research, University of Wisconsin School of Medicine and Public Health, 4235 HSLC, 750 Highland Avenue, Madison, WI 53705, USA
* Corresponding author.
E-mail address: kakumanu@wisc.edu

have shown that both asthma exacerbations and school absenteeism due to asthma have significantly decreased in the past decade (**Fig. 1**). During this time, children with asthma were more likely to participate in programs addressing asthma education and more likely to receive an asthma action plan (AAP). Nevertheless, asthma exacerbations remain frequent and result in significant health care utilization: One in 6 children with asthma (16.7%) are seen in the emergency room (ER) for their asthma symptoms each year and 1 in 20 (4.7%) result in hospitalizations.[1]

Decreases in asthma exacerbation rates in school children with asthma have also been accompanied by decreases in school absenteeism. However, recently published CDC data show that nearly half of all children with asthma report missing 1 or more school days each year due to asthma.[1] These absences can significantly impact a child's school performance, and especially in vulnerable populations, lead to a cycle of lifelong academic achievement.[2] In addition, children from low-income families are at a greater risk of impaired access to health care and health insurance and experience a higher degree of fragmented school health resources.

Since 2001, there has been an increasing public awareness of the need for improved asthma control and pediatric asthma care coordination. Advances in asthma guidelines and clinical trials have provided clinicians with increasing tools to assess asthma risk and control, whereas clinical trials have guided clinicians on the best practices and treatments for patients with poor asthma control. In addition, federal and local agencies have advocated for increased patient education and self-management tools, such as the widespread use of AAPs. 2013 CDC data shows that more children receive AAPs (39% in 2003 vs 51% in 2013) and more children receive asthma education, either in clinics or in school, as compared to prior decades.[1]

Despite these system-wide initiatives to improve asthma awareness and self-management, children with asthma lack consistent use of daily controller medications. In fact, CDC data indicate that only 30% of children with asthma use their asthma controller medications every day, whereas 67% report using their rescue medications within the past 3 months. Future work, state and federal legislation, and local school district policies will need to address interventions that improve the use of asthma controller medications and improve care coordination programs that advocate the

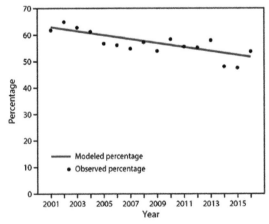

Fig. 1. The percentage of asthma exacerbations in children ages 0 to 17 and school absences as reported by the CDC. (*From* Zahran HS, Bailey CM, Damon SA, et al. Vital signs: asthma in children - United States, 2001-2016. MMWR Morb Mortal Wkly Rep 2018; 67(5):152; with permission.)

daily use of asthma controller medications. Schools, especially those that are staffed by a full-time registered nurse, can be powerful health care partners in addressing this need, both in their ability to consistently deliver asthma medication and in their resources to provide asthma education and asthma monitoring.

HOW SCHOOLS CAN IMPROVE PEDIATRIC ASTHMA CARE COORDINATION

Data have shown that schools can be powerful institutions to affect behavioral change in children with asthma.[3] The positive impact of school nurses on chronic disease management is well known and has been associated with significant improvements in immunization rates, vision screening, asthma exacerbation rates, and decreases in school absences for asthma.[4] Even though school nurses provide important community-based health care to nearly 50 million public school children, they are often not included in collaborative health partnerships. Recent efforts, such as the establishment of the widely endorsed School-based Asthma Management Program (SAMPRO), have supported a greater integration of schools and school nurses into the pediatric asthma care team.[5]

Several studies have supported the use of school-centered asthma programs to improve the delivery of asthma medications and AAPs to schools.[6–10] Schools, especially when staffed by full-time registered school nurses, provide an infrastructure already in place within a child's daily community to monitor their chronic health condition. Programs that have harnessed the use of school nurses to improve asthma management have been shown to decrease asthma exacerbations and improve school attendance. In particular, 2 recently published programs, one that used a school-based telemedicine intervention and another that facilitated asthma care with community-based, school asthma liaisons, have reported promising results.

In a recently published study, four hundred elementary school children, identified with physician-diagnosed asthma, were enrolled in a randomized controlled trial evaluating the effect of regular school-based telemedicine visits to establish and monitor an asthma treatment plan.[10] The treatment plan was initiated at the onset of the school year with a telemedicine clinician who recommended a treatment plan that was delivered through directly observed therapy (DOT) in the school health office and coordinated with the child's primary care provider (PCP). This care was compared with children who received enhanced usual care consisting of a guideline-based symptoms assessment, asthma education, and recommendations for a treatment plan sent to the PCP. The primary outcome, number of symptom-free days, significantly improved in the school-based telemedicine group (11.6 in school-based group vs 10.9 in an enhanced usual care group within a 14-day period), and importantly, ER visits and hospitalizations were significantly reduced (7% in the school-based telemedicine group vs 15% in the usual care group odds ratio 0.52; 95% confidence interval 0.32–0.84). The study also showed promising feasibility of a school-based intervention in an underresourced district. In fact, the study showed significant results in an urban, low-income elementary school that was not staffed with a full-time school nurse, resulting in only 82% of children eligible for DOT actually receiving it.[10] Other studies, using a similar intervention to deliver asthma education without DOT, showed no statistically significant differences in symptom-free days reported, suggesting that DOT by the school nurse is a key aspect of the effective intervention.[11] Further studies are needed to investigate best practices in disseminating and implementing similar tools for school-based management of asthma, and increased advocacy is needed to support adequate funding of these initiatives for all eligible children.

Another well-established program involves the use of a multidisciplinary asthma care team to provide intensive asthma case management, asthma education, and care coordination facilitated by community-based bilingual asthma educators.[6,12] The program, implemented in a large urban, low-income school district in Denver, Colorado, began with strong stakeholder engagement and support from school administrators, school nurses, clinicians, patients, and their families. Key aspects of the program involved training of this adjunct asthma educator/counselor to review asthma and inhaler education, engaging families to serve as their own health care advocates within the traditional and school health systems, establishing professional development for the school nurses in asthma management for sustainability, and providing a system to coordinate the delivery of AAPs and evaluate asthma control. Two hundred fifty-two children receiving free and reduced lunch were recruited from Denver Public Schools into the Step-Up Asthma program. They participated in a comprehensive education program during the school day and a minimum of 4 care coordination services with the asthma counselors who, when needed, coordinated care with clinicians. Children in the program reported statistically significant reductions in asthma exacerbations, urgent care visits, and school absences.[12]

In addition to interventions using school-based telemedicine and community-based workers, previously implemented programs, such as mobile school-based health clinics (SBHC) and innovative Breathmobile programs, have increased access to asthma care and shown similar statistically significant improvements in asthma exacerbation rates, school absenteeism, and asthma control, particularly for high-risk, low-income populations.[13–15] SBHCs offer the additional benefit of providing an infrastructure for the delivery and integration of a wide spectrum of chronic health disease services. It is important to emphasize that each community may need to develop their own school-based implementation practice that is best adapted to their individual patient, clinician, and school health populations. Cultural competencies, state and local regulations, school district policy, and staffing of school health resources will impact the availability, funding, and subsequent delivery of an effective school-based asthma program. With these considerations in mind, and after review of the shared aspects common to successful school-based asthma interventions, the American Academy of Allergy, Asthma, and Immunology (AAAAI) in collaboration with the National Association of School Nurses, developed the SAMPRO and have worked with national partners for widespread endorsement and dissemination.[5]

DEVELOPING AN SCHOOL-BASED ASTHMA MANAGEMENT PROGRAM

In 2016, the AAAAI, in collaboration with the National Association of School Nurses, developed an SAMPRO with 4 key components.[5] These components include the following:

1. A Circle of Support described as a coordinated model for communication among patients, families, clinicians, and school nurses (**Fig. 2**);
2. The use of Asthma Management Plans (AMPs) to provide emergency and individualized asthma care in schools;
3. Comprehensive asthma education for patients, families, and schools; and
4. Strategies for reduction of school environmental triggers.[5]

The AMPs include individualized AAPs and a standardized Asthma Emergency Treatment Plan for schools that detail an emergency treatment plans for all students.

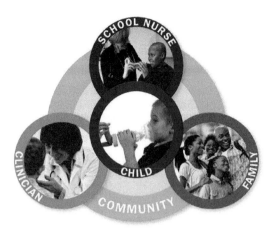

Fig. 2. The SAMPRO advocates for establishing a Circle of Support, consisting of families, clinicians, and school nurses centered on the child with asthma. (*Modified from* American Academy of Allergy Asthma & Immunology. Available at: https://www.aaaai.org/conditions-and-treatments/school-tools/SAMPRO. Accessed January 15, 2019.)

Component One: Circle of Support

The foundation of SAMPRO emanates from establishing a Circle of Support centered on the child with asthma. Building the Circle of Support involves several key steps, including the following:

1. Founding partnerships and pathways of communication around the child among the families, clinicians, and school nurses;
2. Ensuring that clinicians develop individualized AAPs, medications, and complete authorization forms at the initiation of the school year to optimize the monitoring of systems and delivery of asthma medications at schools;
3. Educating school nurses and families with evidence-based asthma education programs to better recognize and self-manage asthma systems; and
4. Reducing communication barriers among all members of the Circle of Support.

It is important to recognize that school-based telemedicine, extended electronic medical record access, and community health workers can all play a role in each of these steps, and the best intervention will depend on the individual needs of each community.

Component Two: Asthma Management Plans

Component 2 involves the use of AMPs, which includes the Asthma Emergency Plan and an AAP for use at home and at school[5] (**Box 1**, **Figs. 3** and **4**). The Asthma Emergency Treatment Plan provides an emergency management plan designed for the child at school with acute asthma symptoms, without an individualized or updated AAP available. The use of the asthma emergency treatment plan by schools allows the delivery of rescue medications for children of high medical necessity and supports the stocking of albuterol in all schools.

In addition to the Asthma Emergency Treatment Plan, SAMPRO advocates the use of an individualized AAP developed for use at home and at school. The SAMPRO AAP (see **Fig. 4**) uses the familiar stoplight algorithm with additional key features. These features include asthma severity, risk for future asthma exacerbations, asthma

---

Box 1
Risk factors for fatal asthma attacks

Asthma history
- Previous severe exacerbation (eg, intubation or intensive care unit admission for asthma)
- Two or more hospitalizations for asthma in the past year
- Three or more emergency department visits for asthma in the past year
- Hospitalization or emergency department visit for asthma in the past month
- Using >2 canisters of short-acting beta2-agonist per month
- Difficulty perceiving asthma symptoms or severity of exacerbations
- Other risk factors: lack of a written AAP, sensitivity to *Alternaria*

Social history
- Low socioeconomic status or inner-city residence
- Illicit drug use
- Major psychosocial problems

Comorbidities
- Cardiovascular disease
- Other chronic lung disease
- Chronic psychiatric disease

Adapted from National Heart, Lung, and Blood Institute (NHLBI). Expert panel report 3: guidelines for the diagnosis and management of asthma, 2007. Available at: https://www.nhlbi.nih.gov/health-topics/guidelines-for-diagnosis-management-of-asthma. Accessed October 12, 2018; with permission.

---

triggers, identification of asthma medications to be administered at school (including the need for preexercise albuterol), parental release of information, and the authorization for a child to self-carry and administer asthma medications.

It is important to recognize that the school nurse is a key health care provider that is based in the school setting. Both clinicians and school nurses need to exchange protected health information in accordance with HIPAA and FERPA privacy laws, local school district policy, and individual health organization legal regulations. The SAMPRO AAP includes a paragraph addressing these privacy concerns with participating entities. Along with the AAP, individual schools may require authorizations for the delivery of medications at schools, and clinicians may need to prescribe additional medications for home and school. In addition, the SAMPRO workforce strongly recommends faxing, the use of secure Web portals, or electronically transmitting AAPs directly from the clinician to the school nurse to facilitate the reliable health information exchange among health care providers.

The implementation of the AAP in school requires that the school nurse receives and processes the forms securely and in a timely manner. SAMPRO strongly advocates for communication infrastructures that facilitate the electronic delivery of AAPs as well as periodic updates of the changes to a child's asthma status, including recent hospitalizations and ER visits, from the clinician to the school nurse. In this manner, the Circle of Support is a living communication framework that facilitates the bidirectional flow of communication that allows the school nurse to share changes in a child's activity or health status with clinicians and facilitates critical elements of asthma care coordination among families, school nurses, and clinicians.

Component Three: Comprehensive Asthma Education

Comprehensive asthma education, particularly programs that engage students, families, clinicians, and schools as an integrated team, has been shown to improve asthma knowledge and self-efficacy.[7,16,17] Furthermore, within the schools, identifying

Assess Severity

- Students at high risk for a fatal attack (see Risk Factors for Fatal Asthma Attacks below) require immediate attention after initial treatment.

- Symptoms and signs suggestive of a more serious exacerbation such as marked breathlessness, inability to speak more than short phrases, use of accessory muscles, or drowsiness should result in initial treatment while immediately calling 911.

- Less severe signs and symptoms can be treated initially with assessment of response to therapy and further steps as listed below.

Initial Treatment

- Inhaled SABA (albuterol) up to two treatments 20 min apart of either :
  - 2–6 puffs by metered-dose inhaler (MDI) and spacer (when available)
  - Nebulizer treatments with albuterol sulfate inhalation solution 0.083% (2.5 mg/3 mL).

Key: SABA: short acting beta2-agonist (quick relief inhaler)

Good Response	Incomplete Response	Poor Response
No wheezing, cough, or dyspnea (assess tachypnea in young children).	Persistent wheezing, cough, and dyspnea (assess tachypnea).	Marked wheezing, cough, and dyspnea.
• Contact parent/guardian for follow-up instructions and further management. • May continue inhaled SABA every 3 to 4 h for 24–48 h. • Return to class and recheck later.	• Continue inhaled SABA as listed under initial treatment above. • Contact parent/guardian, who should follow up urgently with health care provider. • If parent/guardian not available, call 911.	• Repeat inhaled SABA immediately. • If distress is severe and nonresponsive to initial treatment, call 911, then call parent/guardian.

To Hospital Emergency Department

Fig. 3. Asthma Emergency Treatment Plan for the child with acute asthma symptoms at school. This plan is developed to treat urgent asthma symptoms for the child without an updated individualized AAP available at school. SABA, short-acting beta2-agonist. (*Adapted from* National Heart, Lung, and Blood Institute (NHLBI). Expert panel report 3: guidelines for the diagnosis and management of asthma, 2007. Available at: https://www.nhlbi.nih.gov/health-topics/guidelines-for-diagnosis-management-of-asthma. Accessed October 11, 2018; with permission.)

asthma champions throughout the school system, including school nurses, teachers, administrators, and custodial staff, can help to improve dissemination of asthma education and improve programmatic success.[3,18,19]

Component 3 involves the development of a comprehensive education plan for families and schools that identifies the child with asthma, recognizes asthma symptoms, evaluates asthma control with validated tools, and uses best practices in care coordination, communication, and asthma management within the home and school. School health officials and school nurses can promote the use of formal education

AAAAI American Academy of
       Allergy Asthma & Immunology

Name: Birthdate:

Asthma Severity: ☐ Intermittent   ☐ Mild Persistent   ☐ Moderate Persistent   ☐ Severe Persistent
                        ☐ He/she has had many or severe asthma attacks/exacerbations

---

☺ **Green Zone**   Have the child take these medicines every day, even when the child feels well.

Always use a spacer with inhalers as directed.
Controller Medicine(s): _____

Controller Medicine(s) Given in School: _____
Rescue Medicine: Albuterol/Levalbuterol _____ puffs every four hours as needed
Exercise Medicine: Albuterol/Levalbuterol _____ puffs 15 minutes before activity as needed

---

☺ **Yellow Zone**   Begin the sick treatment plan if the child has a cough, wheeze, shortness of breath, or tight chest. Have the
                        child take all of these medicines when sick.

Rescue Medicine: Albuterol/Levalbuterol _____ puffs every 4 hours as needed
Controller Medicine(s):
☐ Continue Green Zone medicines: _____
☐ Add: _____
_____
☐ Change: _____
If the child is in the **yellow** zone more than **24** hours or is getting worse, follow **red** zone and call the doctor right away!

⊗ **Red Zone**   If breathing is hard and fast, ribs sticking out, trouble walking, talking, or sleeping.
                                                Get Help Now

Take rescue medicine(s) now
Rescue Medicine: Albuterol/Levalbuterol _____ puffs every _____
Take: _____

If the child is not better right away, call 911
Please call the doctor any time the child is in the red zone.

Asthma Triggers: (List)

School Staff: Follow the Yellow and Red Zone plans for rescue medicines according to asthma symptoms.
Unless otherwise noted, the only controllers to be administered in school are those listed as "given in school" in the green zone.
☐ Both the asthma provider and the parent feel that the child _may carry and self-administer their inhalers_
☐ School nurse agrees with student self-administering the inhalers

Asthma Provider Printed Name and Contact Information:	Asthma Provider Signature:
	Date:

Parent/Guardian: I give written authorization for the medications listed in the action plan to be administered in school by the nurse or other school members as appropriate. I consent to communication between the prescribing health care provider/clinic, the school nurse, the school medical advisor and school-based health clinic providers necessary for asthma management and administration of this medication.

Parent/guardian signature:	School Nurse Reviewed:
Date:	Date:

Please send a signed copy back to the provider listed above.

Fig. 4. The SAMPRO AAP for use at home or at school. (*Courtesy of* American Academy of Allergy Asthma & Immunology, Milwaukee, WI.)

programs, such as the American Lung Association's Open Airways for Schools, Kickin' Asthma, Iggy and the Inhalers, and Fight Asthma Now, to improve self-efficacy and knowledge of asthma management and understanding by students and school staff.[16,17,20,21] In this way, the school nurse serves as a health care provider and advocate for children in school and supports recognition and treatment of asthma symptoms at the time of onset. Links to these and other programs are available in the SAMPRO toolkit.

Component Four: Environmental Asthma Management

Component 4 advocates for the reduction of asthma triggers found within the school environment. It is well recognized that environmental exposures can influence the development of asthma symptoms, and school poses unique triggers that may affect a child's asthma.[22,23] In addition, specific triggers may differ depending on the school's setting and resources. For example, data from school-based studies in the inner city have shown that mouse allergen is present in significant levels in the school environment and may be associated with increased asthma morbidity.[24,25] Other studies have indicated that individual schools may expose children to higher levels of air pollutants based on proximity to high-density traffic, idling school buses, poor ventilation, and suboptimal building ventilation and maintenance.[26] Current evidence and expert consensus support allergen removal, pest management, and mitigation of air pollutants in the school environment via multifaceted interventions.[24,27]

Recent data have also suggested that variations in school endotoxin exposure may potentially influence children with asthma.[28] Current studies are limited and have primarily involved the inner-city population. Given that the school microbiome is likely affected by student population, urban versus rural settings, climate, and components within individual buildings, future work is needed to establish the relationship between school microbiomes and pediatric asthma.

The Environmental Protection Agency has developed the Indoor Quality Tools program (http://www.epa.gov/iaq/schools/managingasthma.html) to empower schools and families to mitigate pertinent allergen and pollutant exposures within their individual school environments. Using this resource, schools can access walk through checklists, mobile apps, and relevant links to help identify strategies to reduce exposure to air pollutants, such as school bus diesel exhaust, and to use integrated pest management tools as well as mold and mite reduction programs.

SCHOOL-BASED ASTHMA MANAGEMENT PROGRAM: DISSEMINATION AND IMPLEMENTATION

To promote the use of the program, the SAMPRO workforce and the AAAAI have committed resources to develop comprehensive recommendations in its white paper and the development of the SAMPRO toolkit to establish program efficacy.

The SAMPRO toolkit (available at http://aaaai.sampro.org/), constructed in collaboration with the University of Wisconsin HIPxchange program, contains additional key resources, online learning, and downloadable electronic forms of the Asthma Emergency Plan, the AAP, and the Supplementary School Treatment Form in English and Spanish. This toolkit is a powerful dissemination tool that provides users with tangible resources for dissemination and implementation of SAMPRO in local communities, including slide sets with and without narration, videos to teach inhaler techniques, and links to educational and other online tools developed outside the SAMPRO workforce. Checklists for each member of the Circle of Support are available to promote the pediatric asthma care coordination that is the bedrock of the Circle of Support. Recent advances also include the creation of maintenance of certification (MOC) part II and part IV activities for physicians, clinic nurses, and school health nurses.

SUMMARY AND FUTURE CONSIDERATIONS

Childhood asthma remains the most common cause for school absences and is marked by frequent and episodic exacerbations. Schools, particularly those with full-time registered school nurses, provide an established system to deliver health care and patient education and improve monitoring of asthma symptoms. SAMPRO is a widely endorsed school health program that promotes an integrated approach to coordinate pediatric asthma care among clinicians, families, and school nurses.

In parallel to the development of the white paper and toolkit, the SAMPRO workforce and the AAAAI have supported state and federal legislation to support government funding and financial incentives to support school-based asthma care. It is important to recognize that sustainability of SAMPRO will depend on schools having adequate financial resources to maintain funding for school health that coordinate care with clinicians, the stocking of asthma rescue and controller medications, and infrastructure for training of school personnel on asthma management. Future efforts should focus on standardizing requirements for the exchange of health care information among families, schools, and clinicians and to establish a system of standardized data collection to assess health and educational for children with asthma.

REFERENCES

1. Zahran HS, Bailey CM, Damon SA, et al. Vital signs: asthma in children - United States, 2001-2016. MMWR Morb Mortal Wkly Rep 2018;67:149–55.
2. Michael SL, Merlo CL, Basch CE, et al. Critical connections: health and academics. J Sch Health 2015;85(11):740–58.
3. Cicutto L, Gleason M, Szefler SJ. Establishing school-centered asthma programs. J Allergy Clin Immunol 2014;134(6):1223–30 [quiz: 1231].
4. American Academy of Pediatrics Council on School Health, Magalnick H, Mazyck D. Role of the school nurse in providing school health services. Pediatrics 2008;121(5):1052–6.
5. Lemanske RF Jr, Kakumanu S, Shanovich K, et al. Creation and implementation of SAMPRO: a school-based asthma management program. J Allergy Clin Immunol 2016;138(3):711–23.
6. Liptzin DR, Gleason MC, Cicutto LC, et al. Developing, implementing, and evaluating a school-centered asthma program: step-up asthma program. J Allergy Clin Immunol Pract 2016;4(5):972–9.e1.
7. Coffman JM, Cabana MD, Yelin EH. Do school-based asthma education programs improve self-management and health outcomes? Pediatrics 2009; 124(2):729–42.
8. Halterman JS, Szilagyi PG, Fisher SG, et al. Randomized controlled trial to improve care for urban children with asthma: results of the School-Based Asthma Therapy trial. Arch Pediatr Adolesc Med 2011;165(3):262–8.
9. Kaferle JE, Wimsatt LA. A team-based approach to providing asthma action plans. J Am Board Fam Med 2012;25(2):247–9.
10. Frey SM, Halterman JS. Improving asthma care by building bridges across inpatient, outpatient, and community settings. JAMA Pediatr 2017;171(11):1043–4.
11. Perry TT, Halterman JS, Brown RH, et al. Results of an asthma education program delivered via telemedicine in rural schools. Ann Allergy Asthma Immunol 2018; 120(4):401–8.
12. Gleason M, Cicutto L, Haas-Howard C, et al. Leveraging partnerships: families, schools, and providers working together to improve asthma management. Curr Allergy Asthma Rep 2016;16(10):74.
13. Allison MA, Crane LA, Beaty BL, et al. School-based health centers: improving access and quality of care for low-income adolescents. Pediatrics 2007;120(4): e887–94.

14. Liao O, Morphew T, Amaro S, et al. The Breathmobile: a novel comprehensive school-based mobile asthma care clinic for urban underprivileged children. J Sch Health 2006;76(6):313–9.
15. Morphew T, Scott L, Li M, et al. Mobile health care operations and return on investment in predominantly underserved children with asthma: the breathmobile program. Popul Health Manag 2013;16(4):261–9.
16. Mosnaim GS, Li H, Damitz M, et al. Evaluation of the Fight Asthma Now (FAN) program to improve asthma knowledge in urban youth and teenagers. Ann Allergy Asthma Immunol 2011;107(4):310–6.
17. Bruzzese JM, Markman LB, Appel D, et al. An evaluation of Open Airways for Schools: using college students as instructors. J Asthma 2001;38(4):337–42.
18. Cicutto L, Shocks D, Gleason M, et al. Creating district readiness for implementing evidence-based school-centered asthma programs: Denver Public Schools as a Case Study. NASN Sch Nurse 2016;31(2):112–8.
19. Bruzzese JM, Evans D, Kattan M. School-based asthma programs. J Allergy Clin Immunol 2009;124(2):195–200.
20. Mickel CF, Shanovich KK, Evans MD, et al. Evaluation of a school-based asthma education protocol: iggy and the inhalers. J Sch Nurs 2017;33(3):189–97.
21. Magzamen S, Patel B, Davis A, et al. Kickin' Asthma: school-based asthma education in an urban community. J Sch Health 2008;78(12):655–65.
22. Gold DR, Adamkiewicz G, Arshad SH, et al. NIAID, NIEHS, NHLBI, and MCAN Workshop Report: the indoor environment and childhood asthma-implications for home environmental intervention in asthma prevention and management. J Allergy Clin Immunol 2017;140(4):933–49.
23. Maas T, Kaper J, Sheikh A, et al. Mono and multifaceted inhalant and/or food allergen reduction interventions for preventing asthma in children at high risk of developing asthma. Cochrane Database Syst Rev 2009;(3):CD006480.
24. Matsui EC, McCormack MC. Small steps toward asthma-friendly school environments. JAMA Pediatr 2017;171(1):13–4.
25. Sheehan WJ, Permaul P, Petty CR, et al. Association between allergen exposure in inner-city schools and asthma morbidity among students. JAMA Pediatr 2017; 171(1):31–8.
26. Naja AS, Permaul P, Phipatanakul W. Taming asthma in school-aged children: a comprehensive review. J Allergy Clin Immunol Pract 2018;6(3):726–35.
27. Matsui EC, Perzanowski M, Peng RD, et al. Effect of an integrated pest management intervention on asthma symptoms among mouse-sensitized children and adolescents with asthma: a randomized clinical trial. JAMA 2017;317(10): 1027–36.
28. Lai PS, Sheehan WJ, Gaffin JM, et al. School endotoxin exposure and asthma morbidity in inner-city children. Chest 2015;148(5):1251–8.

New Directions in Pediatric Asthma

Leonard B. Bacharier, MD[a], Theresa W. Guilbert, MD, MS[b,c],*

KEYWORDS

- Asthma • Adherence • Adolescent • Antibacterial agents • Biologics
- Environmental exposures • Inner-city • Lung function

KEY POINTS

- Respiratory viral infections in early life and the development of early allergic sensitization are strongly associated with the inception and persistence of early onset asthma.
- Important areas of prevention investigation include the potential diversification of microbiota through use of pharmaceutical products containing protective bacteria and the use of an asthma biological therapy in early life by reducing or blocking immunoglobulin E or cytokine responses and potentially the response to viral exposure.
- Preschool-aged children with a history of recurrent wheezing, with an increased risk to develop asthma show reduction of disease morbidity with the use of a daily inhaled corticosteroid.
- Further characterization of phenotypes/endotypes and discovery of new biomarkers would allow personalization of therapy and development of new treatment strategies in the future.
- Treatment with high-dose inhaled corticosteroid plus a long-acting beta-agonist, leukotriene modifier, theophylline, anticholinergics, biological therapies, and/or prolonged use of oral corticosteroids are used to achieve control in children with severe asthma.

Disclosure Statement: Dr L.B. Bacharier reports grants from NIH; consultancy and lecture fees from GlaxoSmithKline, Genentech/Novartis, Teva, AstraZeneca, Sanofi/Regeneron, and Boehringer Ingelheim; has received lecture fees from and is on the scientific advisory board for Merck; is on the DBV Technologies data safety monitoring board; has received honoraria for Continuing Medical Education (CME) program development from WebMD/Medscape; is on the advisory boards for Vectura and Circassia; and has received research support from Vectura and Sanofi. T.W. Guilbert reports grants from NIH and Sanofi/Regeneron; personal fees from Teva, GSK, Merck, Regeneron Pharmaceuticals, Novartis/Regeneron, Sanofi/Regeneron, Aviragen, and GSK/Regneron; has consulted for American Board of Pediatrics Pediatric Pulmonary Subboard; and has royalties from UpToDate.

[a] Department of Pediatrics, Washington University School of Medicine in St. Louis, Campus Box 8116, 660 South Euclid Avenue, St Louis, MO 63110, USA; [b] Department of Pediatrics, University of Cincinnati, Cincinnati, OH, USA; [c] Pulmonary Division, Cincinnati Children's Hospital Medical Center, 3333 Burnet Avenue, MLC 7041, Cincinnati, OH 45229, USA
* Corresponding author. 3333 Burnet Avenue, MLC 7041, Cincinnati, OH 45229.
E-mail address: Theresa.Guilbert@cchmc.org

Childhood asthma affects an estimated 6.8 million children in the United States,[1] which places them at significant risk for hospitalizations, emergency room visits, and school absences.[2–4] Management of pediatric asthma is challenging, given the heterogeneous phenotypes that evolve as the child ages. Disease management centers around reducing or eliminating exposure to factors that contribute to disease causation and/or worsen symptoms, such as the reduction of environmental exposure to allergens, pollutants and other environmental factors, the appropriate use of asthma medications, and the effective delivery of education of children and their families and caregivers. However, it is not yet clear how to optimize these approaches, potentially including the customization of therapy by asthma phenotype, and thus several future unmet needs exist.

CHILDHOOD ASTHMA INCEPTION AND PROGRESSION

Asthma is clearly a disorder with both genetic and environmental determinants. Data from longitudinal birth cohorts suggest that infections with, and inappropriate responses to, respiratory viruses, particularly human rhinovirus (HRV) and respiratory syncytial virus,[1–4] as well as the development of early allergic sensitization,[5–7] are strongly associated with the inception and persistence of early onset asthma. The most highly replicated genetic region linked to asthma development is the ORMDL3 locus on chromosome 17q,[8] which seems to be associated with increased susceptibility to human rhinovirus–induced wheezing in early life.[9] Several studies have confirmed that being raised in close proximity to animals in a farm setting is highly protective against the development of asthma,[10,11] blocking the increased susceptibility to early onset asthma conferred by variants in the ORMDL3 locus and reducing the incidence of both atopic and nonatopic wheezing in early life. Most evidence supports the protective effect of farm animals as being mediated by exposure to diverse environmental microbes.[12] Of greater importance was that the same 17q alleles that conferred asthma risk in children with wheezing illnesses in early life also conferred strong protection against early onset asthma in children raised on animal farms.[13] Thus, pharmaceutical products containing protective bacteria, or their products, could prevent early onset asthma by simulating exposure to more diverse microbiota. Moreover, asthma biological therapy may have the potential prevent the development of asthma in susceptible children by reducing or blocking immunoglobulin E (IgE) or cytokine responses related to the allergic immune response and potentially the response to viral exposure. Understanding the effectiveness, safety, and underlying mechanisms of these interventions remains important.

PREVENTION OF PEDIATRIC ASTHMA

Identification of potentially modifiable environmental and host risk factors for asthma development has heralded a shift from disease treatment to primary asthma prevention through alteration of these factors. Recently, a systematic review revealed that smoke exposure at any age is associated with decreased lung function, persistent wheeze, and asthma.[14] Thus, interventions to effectively and substantively reduce exposure to pre- and postnatal smoke may reduce asthma incidence and improve lung function in children. In the westernized lifestyle, increased consumption of a diet dominated by processed foods typically deficient in vitamins and minerals may make growing children more susceptible to atopic disease.[15] This raises the possibility that improving the maternal diet is a low-cost and potentially effective intervention for primary prevention for numerous inflammatory diseases.[16] Maternal prenatal dietary supplementation with vitamin D[17–22] or fish oil[23–25] supplementation have been studied and demonstrate their potential to prevent recurrent wheeze or asthma.

Influence of the gut microbiome on immune development and the manifestations of atopic disease is an ongoing area of study, with evidence that intestinal dysbiosis in early infancy may alter human immune development and that early exposure to a diverse microbial environment is likely protective.[26] These data suggest that modification of environmental bacterial exposures in early life may decrease a child's risk of asthma development through alteration of the child's gastrointestinal and airway microbiomes.

Viral respiratory tract infections are an established risk factor for asthma, suggesting that prevention and modification of these infections may protect children from developing recurrent wheezing and asthma. Prophylactic vaccination,[27,28] antiinflammatory therapies,[29–31] and immunostimulatory agents[32–34] have been studied (with inconsistent results) to assess their effect on prevention or modulation of acute respiratory tract illnesses that may lead to long-term protection from recurrent wheezing and asthma. Further research into modification of the risk and severity of early life infections is essential if asthma prevention is to become a reality.

Immunostimulatory agents, such as bacterial extracts (Ref the RAZI paper), may also have a role in enhancing innate and adaptive immune response to infection by targeting the gut-lung immune axis. It is hoped that ongoing trials and longitudinal birth cohort studies will help identify additional protective strategies, because effective asthma prevention is most likely to require multifactorial approaches.

PRESCHOOL ASTHMA AND ASTHMALIKE SYMPTOMS

For preschool-aged children with a history of recurrent wheezing, but who do not yet meet the definition of persistent disease, and demonstrate increased risk to develop asthma (positive modified asthma predictive index), evidence favors the use of a daily inhaled corticosteroid (ICS)[6,10–12] to reduce disease morbidity. A recent study comparing daily ICS, leukotriene receptor antagonists (LTRA), or intermittent use of ICS used with a short-acting beta-agonist as needed for symptoms in preschool-aged children with mild persistent asthma, daily ICS treatment was found to be the most likely effective therapy in controlling asthma control, particularly in children with aeroallergen sensitization or blood eosinophil counts of at least 300 cells/μL.[14] Alternatively, preschool-aged children who were not sensitized to aeroallergens and had blood eosinophil levels less than 300 cells/μL demonstrated relatively low exacerbation rates with ICS, LTRA, or intermittent ICS treatment. Moreover, therapeutic options beyond Step 2 GINA recommendations in the preschool population have little supporting evidence to date. Treatment of preschool asthma would be advanced with better understanding of the mechanisms of asthmalike symptoms in these children and investigation of alternative therapies. Studies in this age group are needed to determine the efficacy of ICS in combination with other asthma medications (long-acting beta-agonists [LABA], LTRA, and/or long-acting antimuscarinic antagonists) and moderate- to high-dose ICS apart from budesonide. Two large clinical trials that studied the use of azithromycin early in a lower respiratory tract infection (LRTI) have shown efficacy in decreasing the severity or duration of the episode in preschool-aged children with history of recurrent severe LRTIs but not yet persistent disease or receiving controller therapy.[28,29] Further research is needed to establish if children treated with repeated azithromycin treatment are at risk for the development of antibiotic-resistant organisms. Also, the effectiveness of biological therapy in preschool-aged children with significant atopic disease has not yet been studied and may represent an opportunity for early treatment and disease prevention or modification.

OBJECTIVE MEASURES OF LUNG FUNCTION IN PRESCHOOL-AGED CHILDREN

Objective measures of lung function are important in the diagnosis and management of asthma. Spirometry, the pulmonary function testing modality most widely used in asthma, may be difficult for some preschoolers. However, with appropriate coaching and technician training, substantial proportions of 3- and 4-year-old children can complete spirometry.[35] Impulse oscillometry (IOS) is a noninvasive method of measuring lung function during tidal breathing that many preschoolers can perform. Fractional exhaled nitric oxide (FeNO) levels correspond to eosinophilic inflammation and predict responsiveness to corticosteroids. In the future, the degree of bronchodilator response that corresponds to early life asthma should be determined, along with expanding the reference values for key parameters in IOS (eg, area of reactance). Further evidence is needed to understand how elevated FeNO levels distinguish among wheezing phenotypes in infancy and school-aged children and the best clinical use of FeNO.

SCHOOL-AGED CHILDREN WITH ASTHMA

Asthma management encompasses the day-to-day treatment of the disease itself, in addition to management of comorbidities and education of patient and family. The lack of effect of treatment of asymptomatic gastroesophageal reflux on asthma control in children with persistent asthma (REF: Teague WG JAMA) demonstrates the importance of robust clinical trials in examining the effects of treatment of comorbidities in achieving improved asthma outcomes. As mentioned earlier, a child's specific disease phenotype may affect the response to pharmacologic treatment.

Children with an allergic or T2-high phenotype (elevated FeNO, peripheral eosinophilia, elevated allergen-specific IgE or positive skin tests) are more likely to respond to daily ICS than LTRAs. For patients who do not achieve an adequate response to ICS or LTRA, particularly those with a neutrophilic or nonatopic phenotype, treatment with macrolide antibiotics (largely azithromycin) may be considered.[36] However, additional studies are needed to determine the efficacy of, and phenotype responsive to, macrolide treatment for asthma.[37]

For children uncontrolled on low-dose ICSs, evidence supports increasing the ICS dose to the moderate range or adding a second controller medication and continuing low-dose ICS.[38,39] In 161 children, a comparison of 3 step-up strategies (medium-dose ICS, low-dose ICS + LABA, low-dose ICS + LTRA) showed a greater likelihood of a better response to LABA step-up than to LTRA or medium-dose ICS dose.[40] Future topics of exploration should include further refinement of asthma phenotypic differences and underlying comorbid conditions, which may affect response to pharmacologic treatment and the underlying mechanisms that drive this response. This is particularly important for those who do not respond to ICS therapy or do not have underlying atopy.

CHILDREN WITH SEVERE ASTHMA

Severe asthma in childhood is a heterogeneous condition, typically defined as asthma that requires a high level of therapy to achieve control or that may remain uncontrolled despite this level of therapy. Factors that drive this need for increased therapy include poor access to care, underrecognition of symptoms, high exposures to irritants and/or allergens, suboptimal medication adherence, challenging environmental exposures, comorbid conditions, and treatment refractory severe asthma.[8,41,42] Some of these children may have other conditions that mimic the symptoms of asthma. A thorough evaluation and treatment of the most modifiable of these potential contributors is important. If symptoms continue to be uncontrolled despite addressing this assessment, treatment with high-dose ICS plus an LABA, leukotriene modifier, theophylline, biological therapies, and/or prolonged use of oral corticosteroids are used to achieve control.[4,43,44] Anticholinergic and biological therapy could be used to help minimize the adverse effects from steroid use.[4,41,45] Children with severe asthma often benefit from frequent disease monitoring and a multidisciplinary approach.

Further research should include validation of phenotype/endotype clusters in longitudinal studies with exploration of mechanisms that would allow personalization of therapy and development of new treatment strategies. Discovery of new phenotypic biomarkers will allow for improved asthma phenotype identification and improved management in the future.

PERSONALIZED MEDICINE AND PEDIATRIC ASTHMA
Environmental Exposures

Understanding key factors and relationships of biological, physical, and psychosocial environmental characteristics and the impact on asthma control is important. Multiple studies have shown that a child's home and school environments expose them to multiple indoor allergens (eg, mouse, cockroach, and pets), biological matter (eg, endotoxin), and pollutants (eg, nitrogen dioxide), and these exposures are associated with increased asthma morbidity.[46–49] Furthermore, some environmental exposures can either be protective or be a risk factor for asthma depending on exposure timing. Currently, there is a lack of high-quality evidence demonstrating that single component interventions for indoor allergen exposure reduction can improve asthma outcomes.[50] Higher domestic endotoxin levels are also linked to increased asthma prevalence, severity, and exacerbations.[51–55] In contrast, there are data supporting that early endotoxin exposure is associated with a decreased risk of childhood asthma.[43,56,57]

As mentioned previously, the microbiome in early infancy can influence asthma risk and asthma.[58] Environmental microbiome diversity in the school is linked to increased asthma symptom days.[59] Exposure to high levels of pollutants such as ozone, SO_2, NO_2, $PM_{2.5}$ (aerodynamic diameter of 2.5 microns or less), and CO is associated with asthma exacerbations, symptoms, and hospitalizations.[41,60–63] The psychosocial environment, a child's neighborhood socioeconomic status, family relationships, housing quality, and social networks are also significant contributors to asthma morbidity.[42,44,45,64–67]

Moving forward, investigation should focus on critical exposure windows in pregnancy and childhood through cohort studies and randomized trials. Additional evidence is needed to determine the efficacy of specific allergen and other exposure remediation interventions in order to design multifaceted interventions with the best synergistic effects. Law and policy reform are also needed to reduce environmental and social disparities that lead to poor asthma outcomes.

Addressing Poor Adherence to Treatment

Treatment adherence in young children involves several factors, including the child, family, community, and health care system. Although effective asthma control medications exist,[68–71] patient adherence to these medications is low with adherence rates frequently less than 50%.[71–73] Asthma management recommendations are complex, including difficultly following inhalation device instructions, need for daily medication use and monthly refills, identification and avoidance of triggers, recognition of increase symptoms, and need for action.[74] As a result, many children experience uncontrolled symptoms and potentially preventable exacerbations with consequent decreases in their quality of life.[75–77]

Effective interventions to promote treatment adherence involve multiple components, including monitoring, feedback, education, and cognitive/behavioral interventions. Education content usually includes discussion of asthma, triggers, medications, peak flows, inhalation technique, and review of a written asthma action plan. Behavioral techniques include self-management strategies, feedback, and incentive plans.[78] Health care system navigators or community health care works reinforce to families the importance of following their treatment plan resulting in improvements in adherence and asthma control.[79–81] Treatment adherence monitoring and providing feedback to the child and family may lead to improvement in treatment adherence in children,[82–87] ideally leading to improved asthma outcomes.

Additional research is needed to determine the key intervention components and to establish how to implement and sustain these interventions in at-risk communities and families, particularly young children. More investigation is essential to elucidate the impact of child development on treatment effectiveness and treatment adherence.

Inner-City Asthma

The inner city is a well-established and well-studied location that includes children at high risk for high asthma prevalence, severity, and morbidity. Several risk factors contribute to asthma in inner-city populations including black race and Puerto Rican Hispanic ethnicity,[87,88] prematurity,[89–91] obesity,[92–94] specific aeroallergen[95–99] and pollutant exposure,[57,100–103] socioeconomic status,[87,104,105] and psychosocial factors.[106–108] Environmental[109–112] trigger remediation of dust mite, cockroach, and mouse allergens and medical interventions such as guideline-based asthma care and biological therapy have improved outcomes in the inner-city children with asthma.[113,114] Future work targeting the identification and modification of risk factors and the use of novel interventions will be essential to reduce disparities in this high-risk group of children with asthma.

Community-Based and School Partnerships

Reducing the disparity of health outcomes between children with asthma and healthy children will require extending pediatric asthma care beyond traditional medical settings and engaging in successful health partnerships with the community and schools. School-based asthma programs such as SAMPRO have been demonstrated to improve communication and the dissemination of asthma action plans and medications to schools and the children that attend them.[115–120]

Future directions include determining which intervention components are the most effective in improving asthma outcomes and establishment of a system of standardized data collection to assess health and educational for children with asthma. In order to be sustainable, legislation is needed to support government funding and financial incentives to disseminate and maintain school-based asthma care.

SUMMARY

Several new developments have occurred over the last 5 years relevant to the field of pediatric asthma. Despite these substantial advances, there is much more to learn. Multiple essential areas for further exploration and research have been identified in order to continue the quest to improve pediatric asthma outcomes, particularly in vulnerable, high-risk populations.

REFERENCES

1. Beigelman A, Bacharier LB. Early-life respiratory infections and asthma development: role in disease pathogenesis and potential targets for disease prevention. Curr Opin Allergy Clin Immunol 2016;16(2):172–8.
2. Kwong CG, Bacharier LB. Microbes and the role of antibiotic treatment for wheezy lower respiratory tract illnesses in preschool children. Curr Allergy Asthma Rep 2017;17(5):34.
3. Lemanske RF Jr, Jackson DJ, Gangnon RE, et al. Rhinovirus illnesses during infancy predict subsequent childhood wheezing. J Allergy Clin Immunol 2005; 116(3):571–7.
4. Kusel MM, de Klerk NH, Kebadze T, et al. Early-life respiratory viral infections, atopic sensitization, and risk of subsequent development of persistent asthma. J Allergy Clin Immunol 2007;119(5):1105–10.
5. Illi S, von Mutius E, Lau S, et al. Perennial allergen sensitisation early in life and chronic asthma in children: a birth cohort study. Lancet 2006;368(9537):763–70.
6. Simpson A, Tan VY, Winn J, et al. Beyond atopy: multiple patterns of sensitization in relation to asthma in a birth cohort study. Am J Respir Crit Care Med 2010;181(11):1200–6.
7. Gergen PJ, Togias A. Inner city asthma. Immunol Allergy Clin North Am 2015; 35(1):101–14.
8. Demenais F, Margaritte-Jeannin P, Barnes KC, et al. Multiancestry association study identifies new asthma risk loci that colocalize with immune-cell enhancer marks. Nat Genet 2018;50(1):42–53.
9. Caliskan M, Bochkov YA, Kreiner-Moller E, et al. Rhinovirus wheezing illness and genetic risk of childhood-onset asthma. N Engl J Med 2013;368(15):1398–407.
10. Riedler J, Braun-Fahrlander C, Eder W, et al. Exposure to farming in early life and development of asthma and allergy: a cross-sectional survey. Lancet 2001;358(9288):1129–33.
11. Fuchs O, Genuneit J, Latzin P, et al. Farming environments and childhood atopy, wheeze, lung function, and exhaled nitric oxide. J Allergy Clin Immunol 2012; 130(2):382–8.e6.
12. Ege MJ, Mayer M, Normand AC, et al. Exposure to environmental microorganisms and childhood asthma. N Engl J Med 2011;364(8):701–9.
13. Loss GJ, Depner M, Hose AJ, et al. The early development of wheeze. Environmental determinants and genetic susceptibility at 17q21. Am J Respir Crit Care Med 2016;193(8):889–97.
14. Belgrave DCM, Granell R, Turner SW, et al. Lung function trajectories from preschool age to adulthood and their associations with early life factors: a retrospective analysis of three population-based birth cohort studies. Lancet Respir Med 2018;6(7):526–34.
15. Thomas D. A study on the mineral depletion of the foods available to us as a nation over the period 1940 to 1991. Nutr Health 2003;17(2):85–115.
16. Devereux G. The increase in the prevalence of asthma and allergy: food for thought. Nat Rev Immunol 2006;6(11):869–74.
17. Camargo CA, Rifas-Shiman SL, Litonjua AA, et al. Maternal intake of vitamin D during pregnancy and risk of recurrent wheeze in children at 3 y of age. Am J Clin Nutr 2007;85(3):788–95.
18. Devereux G, Litonjua AA, Turner SW, et al. Maternal vitamin D intake during pregnancy and early childhood wheezing. Am J Clin Nutr 2007;85(3):853–9.

19. Chawes BL, Bønnelykke K, Stokholm J, et al. Effect of vitamin D3 supplementation during pregnancy on risk of persistent wheeze in the offspring: a randomized clinical trial. JAMA 2016;315(4):353–61.

20. Litonjua AA, Carey VJ, Laranjo N, et al. Effect of prenatal supplementation with vitamin D on asthma or recurrent wheezing in offspring by age 3 years: the VDAART randomized clinical trial. JAMA 2016;315(4):362–70.

21. Wolsk HM, Harshfield BJ, Laranjo N, et al. Vitamin D supplementation in pregnancy, prenatal 25(OH)D levels, race, and subsequent asthma or recurrent wheeze in offspring: secondary analyses from the vitamin D antenatal asthma reduction trial. J Allergy Clin Immunol 2017;140(5):1423–9.e5.

22. Wolsk HM, Chawes BL, Litonjua AA, et al. Prenatal vitamin D supplementation reduces risk of asthma/recurrent wheeze in early childhood: a combined analysis of two randomized controlled trials. PLoS One 2017;12(10):e0186657.

23. Gunaratne AW, Makrides M, Collins CT. Maternal prenatal and/or postnatal n-3 long chain polyunsaturated fatty acids (LCPUFA) supplementation for preventing allergies in early childhood. Cochrane Database Syst Rev 2015;(7):CD010085.

24. Hansen S, Strøm M, Maslova E, et al. Fish oil supplementation during pregnancy and allergic respiratory disease in the adult offspring. J Allergy Clin Immunol 2017;139(1):104–11.e4.

25. Bisgaard H, Stokholm J, Chawes BL, et al. Fish oil-derived fatty acids in pregnancy and wheeze and asthma in offspring. N Engl J Med 2016;375(26):2530–9.

26. Cahenzli J, Köller Y, Wyss M, et al. Intestinal microbial diversity during early-life colonization shapes long-term IgE levels. Cell Host Microbe 2013;14(5):559–70.

27. Blanken MO, Rovers MM, Molenaar JM, et al. Respiratory syncytial virus and recurrent wheeze in healthy preterm infants. N Engl J Med 2013;368(19):1791–9.

28. Scheltema NM, Nibbelke EE, Pouw J, et al. Respiratory syncytial virus prevention and asthma in healthy preterm infants: a randomised controlled trial. Lancet Respir Med 2018;6(4):257–64.

29. Beigelman A, Mikols CL, Gunsten SP, et al. Azithromycin attenuates airway inflammation in a mouse model of viral bronchiolitis. Respir Res 2010;11:90.

30. Beigelman A, Isaacson-Schmid M, Sajol G, et al. Randomized trial to evaluate azithromycin's effects on serum and upper airway IL-8 levels and recurrent wheezing in infants with respiratory syncytial virus bronchiolitis. J Allergy Clin Immunol 2015;135(5):1171–8.e1.

31. Zhou Y, Bacharier LB, Isaacson-Schmid M, et al. Azithromycin therapy during respiratory syncytial virus bronchiolitis: upper airway microbiome alterations and subsequent recurrent wheeze. J Allergy Clin Immunol 2016;138(4):1215–9.e5.

32. Esposito S, Soto-Martinez ME, Feleszko W, et al. Nonspecific immunomodulators for recurrent respiratory tract infections, wheezing and asthma in children: a systematic review of mechanistic and clinical evidence. Curr Opin Allergy Clin Immunol 2018;18(3):198–209.

33. Razi CH, Harmancı K, Abacı A, et al. The immunostimulant OM-85 BV prevents wheezing attacks in preschool children. J Allergy Clin Immunol 2010;126(4):763–9.

34. Del-Rio-Navarro BE, Espinosa Rosales F, Flenady V, et al. Immunostimulants for preventing respiratory tract infection in children. Cochrane Database Syst Rev 2006;4:CD004974.

35. Kattan M, Bacharier LB, O'Connor GT, et al. Spirometry and impulse oscillometry in preschool children: acceptability and relationship to maternal smoking in pregnancy. J Allergy Clin Immunol Pract 2018;6(5):1596–603.e6.
36. Piacentini G, Peroni D, Bodini A, et al. Azithromycin reduces bronchial hyperresponsiveness and neutrophilic airway inflammation in asthmatic children: a preliminary report. Allergy Asthma Proc 2007;28:194–8.
37. Strunk RC, Bacharier LB, Phillips BR, et al. Azithromycin or montelukast as inhaled corticosteroid-sparing agents in moderate-to-severe childhood asthma study. J Allergy Clin Immunol 2008;122(6):1138–44.e4.
38. Global Initiative for Asthma. Global strategy for asthma management and prevention. Fontana (WI): Global Initative for Asthma organization; 2018.
39. Guidelines for the diagnosis and management of asthma. Available at: https://www.nhlbi.nih.gov/health-topics/guidelines-for-diagnosis-management-of-asthma. Accessed October 12, 2018.
40. Lemanske R, Mauger D, Sorkness C, et al. Step-up therapy for children with uncontrolled asthma receiving inhaled corticosteroids. N Engl J Med 2010;362:975–85.
41. Orellano P, Quaranta N, Reynoso J, et al. Effect of outdoor air pollution on asthma exacerbations in children and adults: systematic review and multilevel meta-analysis. PLoS One 2017;12(3):e0174050.
42. Williams DR, Sternthal M, Wright RJ. Social determinants: taking the social context of asthma seriously. Pediatrics 2009;123(Supplement 3):S174–84.
43. Karvonen AM, Hyvarinen A, Gehring U, et al. Exposure to microbial agents in house dust and wheezing, atopic dermatitis and atopic sensitization in early childhood: a birth cohort study in rural areas. Clin Exp Allergy 2012;42(8):1246–56.
44. Kopel LS, Gaffin JM, Ozonoff A, et al. Perceived neighborhood safety and asthma morbidity in the school inner-city asthma study. Pediatr Pulmonol 2015;50(1):17–24.
45. Mehta AJ, Dooley DP, Kane J, et al. Subsidized housing and adult asthma in Boston, 2010-2015. Am J Public Health 2018;108(8):1059–65.
46. Salo PM, Arbes SJ, Crockett PW, et al. Exposure to multiple indoor allergens in US homes and its relationship to asthma. J Allergy Clin Immunol 2008;121(3):678–84.e2.
47. Kanchongkittiphon W, Gaffin JM, Phipatanakul W. The indoor environment and inner-city childhood asthma. Asian Pac J Allergy Immunol 2014;32(2):103–10.
48. Simons E, Curtin-Brosnan J, Buckley T, et al. Indoor environmental differences between inner city and suburban homes of children with asthma. J Urban Health 2007;84(4):577–90.
49. Permaul P, Hoffman E, Fu C, et al. Allergens in urban schools and homes of children with asthma. Pediatr Allergy Immunol 2012;23(6):543–9.
50. Leas BF, D'Anci KE, Apter AJ, et al. Effectiveness of indoor allergen reduction in asthma management: a systematic review. J Allergy Clin Immunol 2018;141(5):1854–69.
51. Michel O, Kips J, Duchateau J, et al. Severity of asthma is related to endotoxin in house dust. Am J Respir Crit Care Med 1996;154(6 Pt 1):1641–6.
52. Boehlecke B, Hazucha M, Alexis NE, et al. Low-dose airborne endotoxin exposure enhances bronchial responsiveness to inhaled allergen in atopic asthmatics. J Allergy Clin Immunol 2003;112(6):1241–3.

53. Thorne PS, Mendy A, Metwali N, et al. Endotoxin exposure: predictors and prevalence of associated asthma outcomes in the United States. Am J Respir Crit Care Med 2015;192(11):1287–97.

54. Sheehan WJ, Hoffman EB, Fu C, et al. Endotoxin exposure in inner-city schools and homes of children with asthma. Ann Allergy Asthma Immunol 2012;108(6): 418–22.

55. Lai PS, Sheehan WJ, Gaffin JM, et al. School endotoxin exposure and asthma morbidity in inner-city children. Chest 2015;148(5):1251–8.

56. Stein MM, Hrusch CL, Gozdz J, et al. Innate immunity and asthma risk in amish and hutterite farm children. N Engl J Med 2016;375(5):411–21.

57. O'Connor GT, Lynch SV, Bloomberg GR, et al. Early-life home environment and risk of asthma among inner-city children. J Allergy Clin Immunol 2018;141(4): 1468–75.

58. Stokholm J, Blaser MJ, Thorsen J, et al. Maturation of the gut microbiome and risk of asthma in childhood. Nat Commun 2018;9(1):141.

59. Lai PS, Kolde R, Franzosa EA, et al. The classroom microbiome and asthma morbidity in children attending 3 inner-city schools. J Allergy Clin Immunol 2018;141(6):2311–3.

60. Prunicki M, Stell L, Dinakarpandian D, et al. Exposure to NO 2, CO, and PM 2.5 is linked to regional DNA methylation differences in asthma. Clin Epigenetics 2018;10(1):2.

61. Naja A, Phipatanakul W, Permaul P. Taming asthma in school-aged children: a comprehensive review. J Allergy Clin Immunol 2018;6(3):726–35.

62. Pollock J, Shi L, Gimbel RW. Outdoor environment and pediatric asthma: an update on the evidence from North America. Can Respir J 2017;2017.

63. Yoda Y, Takagi H, Wakamatsu J, et al. Acute effects of air pollutants on pulmonary function among students: a panel study in an isolated island. Environ Health Prev Med 2017;22(1):33.

64. Thakur N, Barcelo NE, Borrell LN, et al. Perceived discrimination associated with asthma and related outcomes in minority youth: the GALA II and SAGE II studies. Chest 2017;151(4):804–12.

65. Chen E, Schreier HM. Does the social environment contribute to asthma? Immunol Allergy Clin North Am 2008;28(3):649–64.

66. Beck AF, Huang B, Ryan PH, et al. Areas with high rates of police-reported violent crime have higher rates of childhood asthma morbidity. J Pediatr 2016; 173:175–82.e1.

67. Shamasunder B, Collier-Oxandale A, Blickley J, et al. Community-based health and exposure study around urban oil developments in south Los Angeles. Int J Environ Res Public Health 2018;15(1):138.

68. National Asthma Education Prevention Program (NAEPP). Expert panel report 3 (EPR-3): Guidelines for the diagnosis and managemetn of asthma-summary report 2007. J Allergy Clin Immunol 2007;120(5 Suppl):S94–138.

69. Blake KV. Improving adherence to asthma medications: Current knowledge and future perspectives. Curr Opin Pulm Med 2017;23:62–70.

70. Bauman LJ, Wright E, Leickly EE, et al. Relationship of adherence to pediatric asthma morbidity among inner-city children. Pediatrics 2002;110:e1–7.

71. McQuaid EL, Kopel SJ, Klein RB, et al. Medication adherence in pediatric asthma: reasoning, responsibility, and behavior. J Pediatr Psychol 2003;28: 323–33.

72. Bender B. Nonadherence to asthma treatment: getting unstuck. J Allergy Clin Immunol Pract 2016;4:849–51.

73. Morton RW, Everard ML, Elphick HE. Adherence in childhood asthma: the elephant in the room. Arch Dis Child 2014;99:949–53.
74. Morawska A, Stelzer J, Burgess S. Parenting asthmatic children: Identification of parenting challenges. J Asthma 2008;45:465–72.
75. Walders N, Kopel SJ, Koinis-Mitchell D, et al. Patterns of quick-relief and long-term controller medication use in pediatric asthma. J Pediatr 2005;146:177–82.
76. Otsuki-Clutter M, Sutter M, Ewig J. Promoting adherence to inhaled corticosteroid therapy in patients with asthma. J Clin Outcomes Manag 2011;18:177–82.
77. Gray WN, Netz M, McConville A, et al. Medication adherence in pediatric asthma: a systematic review of the literature. Pediatr Pulmonol 2018;53:668–84.
78. Apter AJ, Morales KH, Han X, et al. A patient advocate to facilitate access and improve communication, care, and outcomes in adults with moderate or severe asthma: rationale, design, and methods of a randomized controlled trial. Contemp Clin Trials 2017;56:34–45.
79. Fox P, Porter PG, Lob SH, et al. Improving asthma-related health outcomes among low-income, multiethnic, school-aged children: results of a demonstration project that combined continuous quality improvement and community health worker strategies. Pediatrics 2007;120:e902–11.
80. Andreae SJ, Andreae LJ, Cherrington AL, et al. Development of a community health worker-delivered cognitive behavioral training intervention for individuals with diabetes and chronic pain. Fam Community Health 2018;41:178–84.
81. Normansell R, Kew KM, Stovold E. Interventions to improve adherence to inhaled steroids for asthma [review]. Cochrane Database Syst Rev 2017;(4):CD012226.
82. Chuenjit W, Engchuan V, Yuenyongviwat A, et al. Achieving good adherence to inhaled corticosteroids after weighing canisters of asthmatic children. F1000Res 2017;6:266.
83. Spaulding SA, Devine KA, Duncan CL, et al. Electronic monitoring and feedback to improve adherence in pediatric asthma. J Pediatr Psychol 2012;37:64–74.
84. Burgess SW, Sly PD, Devadason SG. Providing feedback on adherence increases use of preventative medication by asthmatic children. J Asthma 2010;47:198–201.
85. Wiecha JM, Adams WG, Rybin D, et al. Evaluation of a web-based asthma self-management system: a randomized controlled pilot trial. BMC Pulm Med 2015;15–7.
86. Elias P, Rajan NO, McArthur K, et al. InSpire to promote lung assessment in youth: evolving the self-management paradigms of young people with asthma. Med 2.0 2013;2:e1.
87. Keet CA, McCormack MC, Pollack CE, et al. Neighborhood poverty, urban residence, race/ethnicity, and asthma: rethinking the inner-city asthma epidemic. J Allergy Clin Immunol 2015;135(3):655–62.
88. Akinbami LJ, Moorman JE, Simon AE, et al. Trends in racial disparities for asthma outcomes among children 0 to 17 years, 2001-2010. J Allergy Clin Immunol 2014;134(3):547–53.e5.
89. He H, Butz A, Keet CA, et al. Preterm birth with childhood asthma: the role of degree of prematurity and asthma definitions. Am J Respir Crit Care Med 2015;192(4):520–3.
90. Crump C, Winkleby MA, Sundquist J, et al. Risk of asthma in young adults who were born preterm: a Swedish national cohort study. Pediatrics 2011;127(4):e913–20.

91. Dombkowski KJ, Leung SW, Gurney JG. Prematurity as a predictor of childhood asthma among low-income children. Ann Epidemiol 2008;18(4):290-7.

92. Robbins JM, Benson BJ, Esangbedo IC, et al. Childhood obesity in an inner-city primary care population: a longitudinal study. J Natl Med Assoc 2016;108(3): 158-63.

93. Elliott JP, Harrison C, Konopka C, et al. Pharmacist-led screening program for an inner-city pediatric population. J Am Pharm Assoc (2003) 2015;55(4):413-8.

94. Vo P, Makker K, Matta-Arroyo E, et al. The association of overweight and obesity with spirometric values in minority children referred for asthma evaluation. J Asthma 2013;50(1):56-63.

95. Rosenstreich DL, Eggleston P, Kattan M, et al. The role of cockroach allergy and exposure to cockroach allergen in causing morbidity among inner-city children with asthma. N Engl J Med 1997;336(19):1356-63.

96. Ahluwalia SK, Peng RD, Breysse PN, et al. Mouse allergen is the major allergen of public health relevance in Baltimore city. J Allergy Clin Immunol 2013;132(4): 830-5.e1-2.

97. Torjusen EN, Diette GB, Breysse PN, et al. Dose-response relationships between mouse allergen exposure and asthma morbidity among urban children and adolescents. Indoor Air 2013;23(4):268-74.

98. Pongracic JA, O'Connor GT, Muilenberg ML, et al. Differential effects of outdoor versus indoor fungal spores on asthma morbidity in inner-city children. J Allergy Clin Immunol 2010;125(3):593-9.

99. Ziello C, Sparks TH, Estrella N, et al. Changes to airborne pollen counts across Europe. PLoS One 2012;7(4):e34076.

100. Kattan M, Gergen PJ, Eggleston P, et al. Health effects of indoor nitrogen dioxide and passive smoking on urban asthmatic children. J Allergy Clin Immunol 2007;120(3):618-24.

101. Hansel NN, Breysse PN, McCormack MC, et al. A longitudinal study of indoor nitrogen dioxide levels and respiratory symptoms in inner-city children with asthma. Environ Health Perspect 2008;116(10):1428-32.

102. Liu AH, Babineau DC, Krouse RZ, et al. Pathways through which asthma risk factors contribute to asthma severity in inner-city children. J Allergy Clin Immunol 2016;138(4):1042-50.

103. Ierodiakonou D, Zanobetti A, Coull BA, et al. Ambient air pollution, lung function, and airway responsiveness in asthmatic children. J Allergy Clin Immunol 2016; 137(2):390-9.

104. Milligan KL, Matsui E, Sharma H. Asthma in urban children: epidemiology, environmental risk factors, and the public health domain. Curr Allergy Asthma Rep 2016;16(4):33.

105. Lynch SV, Wood RA, Boushey H, et al. Effects of early-life exposure to allergens and bacteria on recurrent wheeze and atopy in urban children. J Allergy Clin Immunol 2014;134(3):593-601.e2.

106. Shams MR, Bruce AC, Fitzpatrick AM. Anxiety contributes to poorer asthma outcomes in inner-city black adolescents. J Allergy Clin Immunol Pract 2018;6(1): 227-35.

107. Ramratnam SK, Visness CM, Jaffee KF, et al. Relationships among maternal stress and depression, type 2 responses, and recurrent wheezing at age 3 years in low-income urban families. Am J Respir Crit Care Med 2017;195(5): 674-81.

108. Bellin MH, Collins KS, Osteen P, et al. Characterization of Stress in low-income, inner-city mothers of children with poorly controlled asthma. J Urban Health 2017;94(6):814–23.
109. Morgan WJ, Crain EF, Gruchalla RS, et al. Results of a home-based environmental intervention among urban children with asthma. N Engl J Med 2004; 351(11):1068–80.
110. Rabito FA, Carlson JC, He H, et al. A single intervention for cockroach control reduces cockroach exposure and asthma morbidity in children. J Allergy Clin Immunol 2017;140(2):565–70.
111. Pongracic JA, Visness CM, Gruchalla RS, et al. Effect of mouse allergen and rodent environmental intervention on asthma in inner-city children. Ann Allergy Asthma Immunol 2008;101(1):35–41.
112. Matsui EC, Perzanowski M, Peng RD, et al. Effect of an integrated pest management intervention on asthma symptoms among mouse-sensitized children and adolescents with asthma: a randomized clinical trial. JAMA 2017;317(10): 1027–36.
113. Busse WW, Morgan WJ, Gergen PJ, et al. Randomized trial of omalizumab (anti-IgE) for asthma in inner-city children. N Engl J Med 2011;364(11):1005–15.
114. Teach SJ, Gill MA, Togias A, et al. Preseasonal treatment with either omalizumab or an inhaled corticosteroid boost to prevent fall asthma exacerbations. J Allergy Clin Immunol 2015;136(6):1476–85.
115. Lemanske RF Jr, Kakumanu S, Shanovich K, et al. Creation and implementation of SAMPRO: a school-based asthma management program. J Allergy Clin Immunol 2016;138(3):711–23.
116. Liptzin DR, Gleason MC, Cicutto LC, et al. Developing, implementing, and evaluating a school-centered asthma program: step-up asthma program. J Allergy Clin Immunol Pract 2016;4(5):972–9.e1.
117. Coffman JM, Cabana MD, Yelin EH. Do school-based asthma education programs improve self-management and health outcomes? Pediatrics 2009; 124(2):729–42.
118. Halterman JS, Szilagyi PG, Fisher SG, et al. Randomized controlled trial to improve care for urban children with asthma: results of the School-Based Asthma Therapy trial. Arch Pediatr Adolesc Med 2011;165(3):262–8.
119. Kaferle JE, Wimsatt LA. A team-based approach to providing asthma action plans. J Am Board Fam Med 2012;25(2):247–9.
120. Frey SM, Halterman JS. Improving asthma care by building bridges across inpatient, outpatient, and community settings. JAMA Pediatr 2017;171(11): 1043–4.

Moving?

Make sure your subscription moves with you!

To notify us of your new address, find your **Clinics Account Number** (located on your mailing label above your name), and contact customer service at:

Email: journalscustomerservice-usa@elsevier.com

800-654-2452 (subscribers in the U.S. & Canada)
314-447-8871 (subscribers outside of the U.S. & Canada)

Fax number: 314-447-8029

Elsevier Health Sciences Division
Subscription Customer Service
3251 Riverport Lane
Maryland Heights, MO 63043

*To ensure uninterrupted delivery of your subscription, please notify us at least 4 weeks in advance of move.

Printed and bound by CPI Group (UK) Ltd, Croydon, CR0 4YY

03/10/2024

01040400-0014